Fear Is No Longer
My Reality

Fear Is No Longer My Reality

■ ▮ ■

How I Overcame Panic and
Social Anxiety Disorder—and You Can Too

▪ ▮ ▪

Jamie Blyth
with Jenna Glatzer

McGraw-Hill
New York Chicago San Francisco
Lisbon London Madrid Mexico City
Milan New Delhi San Juan Seoul
Singapore Sydney Toronto

1 2 3 4 5 6 7 8 9 0   DOC/DOC   0 9 8 7 6 5 4

ISBN 0-07-144729-6

McGraw-Hill books are available at special quantity discounts to use as premiums and sales promotions, or for use in corporate training programs. For more information, please write to the Director of Special Sales, McGraw-Hill Professional, Two Penn Plaza, New York, NY 10121-2298. Or contact your local bookstore.

This book is printed on recycled, acid-free paper containing a minimum of 50% recycled, de-inked fiber.

Library of Congress Cataloging-in-Publication Data

Blyth, Jamie.
    Fear is no longer my reality : how I overcame panic and social anxiety disorder—and you can too / Jamie Blyth with Jenna Glatzer.— 1st ed.
      p. cm.
    ISBN 0-07-144729-6 (alk. paper)
    1. Blyth, Jamie—Mental health. 2. Panic disorders—Patients—Biography. 3. Social phobia—Patients—Biography. I. Glatzer, Jenna. II. Title.
RC535.B59   2004
616.85'22'0092—dc22

                                              2004016395

To my mother, Rosemary Blyth

Contents

Contents

Acknowledgments

I would not have had a triumph to write about had it not been for the people who've shaped my life and given it meaning.

First and foremost, I thank my mom. Your love has been strong, unconditional, and selfless. You've made everything I've accomplished possible. I am forever in your debt.

Special thanks to my dad for always being there when I needed him, and to my brothers and sister, Bill, John, and Mara, for putting up with me for all these years. I couldn't have grown up with better people, and I cherish the memories we have together.

Uncle John "Rufus" is the man I turn to when I need advice . . . especially about women (which is the advice I need most). You have been immensely giving and supportive to my family and I know I speak for all of us when I thank you, particularly for the much-needed comic relief.

I owe a debt of gratitude to some close friends who, along with my family, have saved my life over the years. Without these friends, this book would not have been possible: Joe Cheff, Brian Loftus,

Brian Musso, Johnny, Nate Rowe, Pam Garfield, Jamie Marconi, Bridget Coyne, Mike Denvir, Clay, Murph, Doug, Billy C., Alexis, Brandon Beavers, Alex Silva, Ryan Jones, Brian Merrion, Jeff Casey, Shoe, Temp Keller, Joe Hartney, Kara, Young Chung, Katie Shean, Colgate, Brian Wardle, Gross, Rich Kingston, Kenny Mac, John Woodhouse, Mike Keefe, Grant, Mash, Scott, Nelly, Lilly, and "The Baron."

Brian, Johnny "J Dog," Tanner, and "Z," you have shown me the meaning of generosity, hospitality, and humility. It would take the remainder of this book to express all you have done for me and how much you mean to me.

Special thanks to Jenna Glatzer, a tremendously talented writer and an even more amazing person and friend. Your effort and skill are enormously appreciated. Thanks for helping to make this book happen.

Thanks to all of my friends from the show and to the great people at ABC and Telepictures for giving me the opportunity to be on *The Bachelorette* and for making the entire experience so amazing.

Nancy Hancock, Michele Pezzuti, and Michael Broussard, I appreciate your support, insight, and belief in this project. Thank you, too, to all of the mental health professionals who contributed to this book.

So many of you have told me about your personal experiences with anxiety and panic and struggle, and I am honored that you felt comfortable sharing your stories with me. They helped inspire this book and reminded me why it was important.

Finally, I thank our military and their families for their bravery in preserving our freedom.

Jamie Blyth

Introduction

For some people, fear makes sense. They feel fear at appropriate times, like when they watch scary movies, hear loud noises in the middle of the night, or when their cars skid on icy roads. But for other people, fear crops up in situations that don't logically warrant it. Take away that icy road and pretend it's a breezy spring day and you're driving six blocks to go out to dinner with an old friend. Nothing scary about that, right? Unless you're one of us.

If you've picked up this book, perhaps you are among the one in nine people struggling with overwhelming anxiety. Did you know there were so many of us?

Maybe there are times in your life when you are so paralyzed by worry that your day-to-day activities halt completely. You roll out of bed and wish you could roll back in. The thought of getting into your car and driving to work sends you into a tailspin. You're afraid that you'll have a panic attack in aisle five of the grocery store, worried about what people will think of you if you fall apart in line at the bank, afraid that you won't get through another day of "faking it" through the racing heart, the dizziness, and the choking terror that arises every time you have to open your mouth in front of a group of people.

I've been there.

Because I spoke about my anxiety on *The Bachelorette* and later on *Oprah* and other talk shows, I've met and corresponded with literally thousands of people who've been there too. Some of them are still "there." And each time someone asked me how I got past my years of panic, I wanted to give more than a one-minute summary. I knew that I could never encapsulate everything I learned and all the strategies I used to get better in the short time I was given to spend with each of these people.

I began writing down all the things I wanted to share. I thought back to the time when panic seemed like an insurmountable wall, and I couldn't see any future beyond it. My self-esteem was shattered. I felt like Humpty Dumpty, broken into a million tiny pieces and unable to put myself back together again. More than anything, I felt hopelessly alone, convinced no one in the world could understand what I was going through.

But there are more than 20 million of us in America alone who *do* understand. According to the American Psychiatric Institute ("Let's Talk Facts About Anxiety Disorders," 1999), anxiety disorder is the most common mental health problem in the United States today. It's not always easy to believe that, though, because so many people are still afraid to talk about it. As pages turned into chapters, my first goal was to provide comfort to those who still feel alone. In this book, I'm going to tell you about how panic engulfed my life and overpowered me. Then I'm going to tell you how I fought back using strength I never believed I had. It is my deep hope that when you are finished reading this book, you will realize there is no reason to be ashamed and that if I can win this fight, you can too.

I have also invited top mental health professionals who specialize in anxiety disorders to help explain what anxiety disorders are, what effects they have, who gets them, and why you can quit beating yourself up for not being able to just "snap out of it." The terror brought on by anxiety disorders is very real. These experts have put a sometimes-complicated topic into words that anyone can understand. If you've wanted to tell someone what you're going through, you might share this book and let the doctors help you explain.

As the book progresses, you will also learn how to beat your anxiety by using coping strategies, visualizations, positive thinking, relaxation techniques, and breathing exercises, as well as how you can find a therapist trained to guide you through your recovery.

I've detailed what worked for me—and what didn't work—so you can see if you'd like to try any of my methods. My "Panic Plan" gives an easy-to-follow map of the steps I used to build myself up and knock the anxiety down.

The anxiety specialists have also shared their advice about tools and techniques that have proven to be effective. We've come a long way in the treatment of anxiety disorders in recent years and now know that there are many forms of therapy, medication, and self-help strategies that work. If you follow the guidelines presented in this book, you can free yourself of severe anxiety and live the life you were meant to live.

Having an anxiety disorder doesn't mean that you're weak, crazy, worthless, or inept. All it means is that you have a hurdle to overcome. If you rise to the challenge, you'll find yourself stronger and more alive than you've ever been before.

When you finish this book, I hope you won't close it thinking about anxiety and worry, but instead, thinking about dreams and possibility. We are not defined by our obstacles, but by our responses to them. Anxiety can be a terrific gift if you allow it to be. It can bring out your personal best and give you the opportunity to show yourself that you are worth fighting for and that you have an unbreakable spirit.

Thank you for picking up my book. I am grateful for the opportunity to share my story with you.

Fear Is No Longer
My Reality

Emerging

The greater the obstacle,
the greater the glory in overcoming it.
—MOLIERE

It was time. I put on my dark pin-striped suit, the first suit I had ever purchased, the same suit that had traveled with me from one end of myself to the other. This was to be a defining moment in my life, a moment that would let me prove that I had emerged from the shadow that had darkened my world for so many years. Either that, or I was going to humiliate myself in front of millions of people and live out my remaining days with a paper bag over my head. Fifty-fifty odds, I figured.

I glanced in the mirror, took a deep breath, cleared my throat of some excess nerves, and walked out the door of my Universal Studios' Hyatt hotel room and through the front lobby. A black stretch limo was waiting for me, shining in the last bits of sunshine. I was on my way to meet a woman named Trista, to be the first man to appear in front of nationwide viewers on ABC's new reality series *The Bachelorette*.

The trip was supposed to take about an hour. Five strangers accompanied me on the ride; these were to be some of the other "suitors" on the show. Each of us would compete to win Trista's heart by charming her on group or solo dates, and she'd eliminate one or more of us each week until just one man was left. We made small talk, but my mind was busy with its own internal monologue. As I stared out the window at the Pacific Ocean, a gamut of thoughts and images washed over me.

There are certain memories that stay forever intact, able to be called up and reexperienced down to the tiniest detail as if they're happening *right now*—especially when you least want them to interfere. As I sat there in that limo, my mind traveled back in time. I felt like I was 19 years old again and in the midst of my first panic attack, a lightning bolt that crashed down on me and split my life in two: before and after. The experience lasted only a minute or so, but in that time, my life changed forever. I didn't yet have a name for the thing that had overtaken my mind and body in that minute; all I knew was that I lived in constant terror of its ever happening again.

The next image I saw was myself in my single dorm room at college, doing anything I could to avoid my intense fear of people and panic. I locked myself in that room for almost a month, hiding out in the darkness, trembling and occasionally erupting in hot tears of desolation. The attacks had gotten so strong that I was usually unable to make it to class, and when I did, I couldn't speak. I told no one what I was going through because it felt shameful to me then.

Panic left a mark on me, a scar. It was a whispering phantom that followed me wherever I went, telling me to give up hope and retreat to the safety of solitude. My world became colorless and the future invisible.

■ ■ ■

According to the American Psychiatric Association: "Anxiety disorders are the most common emotional disorders, annually affecting more than 20 million Americans— or about *one in nine people*."

■ ■ ■

Just a few months earlier, these memories might have stopped me in my tracks. Memories can be powerful triggers, and just thinking about my past panic attacks used to be enough to bring on a new one. I was still vulnerable, but now I knew how to recognize my triggers, and I had a strategy for getting past them. Not long ago, those scary thoughts might have convinced me to tell that driver to pull over and let me out. But not this time. This time, I felt pride. It took every ounce of strength in me just to make it out of that self-imposed prison alive. These flashing images were my proof of success: look how far I had already come. Here I was in California, with no bedroom to run into, no door to lock behind me, nowhere to hide. I was going through with this adventure, for better or worse.

The driver snapped me back to the present when he told us we were five minutes away from the house. The sun had crept off while I was daydreaming; night had set in. Off to my left, I noticed an enormous mansion ablaze in a circle of light, shining high up in the hills like a bright white moon. That's when "or worse" came a little sooner than I had hoped.

My heart pounded in my chest, butterflies seized my stomach, and my lungs tightened as I gasped for air. My internal voice went off in a million directions. *What kind of impression will I make? How should I introduce myself? Will I hold up or break down crying with a panic attack in front of the camera, in front of millions? What was I thinking? I'm not ready for this! Just three years ago, I couldn't even go on a date and now I'm supposed to compete for a woman's affections on national television?*

I sat rigidly in my seat, bracing for the inevitable. We approached the mansion and I thought I was going to lose it. I didn't even know if I would be able to utter a word. We pulled up to the front drive and an attractive blonde sat on the steps about 20 feet away, surrounded by a multitude of television cameras, boom mikes, blindingly intense lights, and crew members. Jason, the director, greeted me warmly and told me that the limo driver would open my door for me, which would be my cue to walk out and talk to Trista.

Sure, just make casual conversation while all of America listens in—while my throat is closed down and it feels like a boa constrictor has wrapped itself around my ribcage and begun to squeeze out the last bit of oxygen left. Simple.

"Wait ... wait!" I called. But it was too late. Why did I have to be first? Couldn't we do a practice run, or at least let me walk around a little and get used to the place?

■ ■ ■

I was sitting right next to him and he just looked a little sweaty and scared. At that point, I didn't know anything about any sort of anxiety condition, so I figured it was just basic nerves from being on the show. I took his pulse. I learned through my job as a firefighter that sometimes if you take someone's pulse and reassure them that they're healthy, although you're not really doing anything medically, it's somehow soothing. His pulse was fast, but I think probably everyone's pulse was a little fast. At that point, no one really knew the extent of what Jamie may have been going through. We all just figured he had the same nervousness as we did. No one could particularly understand it because he seemed at first glance to be a pretty self-confident person who really would have no cause for nerves.

—Ryan Sutter (a competing Bachelor on *The Bachelorette*)

■ ■ ■

Nervous chatter overtook me, and I looked to these new acquaintances for support. Ryan told me, "Man, I thought I was going to be the only person who was this nervous." He reassured me that I wasn't alone.

I felt electric inside, buzzing with adrenaline and fear. I again listened to the voice inside, counseling me, "Be brave. You have no reason to panic. You've felt this way a million times and come out on top. This is going to be fun, a challenge, something to look forward to. Get tough."

I said a silent prayer, begging God to give me strength.

The driver walked my way. My energy ran so high I thought I might explode, but the fear mixed with elation, almost giddiness. If I could just get through this next 30 seconds, I could do anything. My determination returned, and I decided that whatever had gotten me to this place was going to carry me through. I was already smiling when the driver opened the door. My ridiculously white teeth made their entrance on the show before I did.

"Men die of fright and live of confidence." I whispered these words of Thoreau's to myself and squared my shoulders.

Stepping out of the car, I walked with unsteady legs through a haze of lights and cameras, focusing on Trista as I approached her. Her beaming smile was a welcome sight, and I summoned the strength to take those 15 steps.

"Hi Trista," I said. "I'm Jamie. It's nice to meet you." Then I told her she looked great and kissed her on the cheek.

Simple.

Walking past her, I glanced back with a smile, knowing that I did a good job, that the cameras couldn't capture the "reality" of what was happening inside. This was victory. This was my Mount Everest, and I felt as if I had just summitted in shorts.

■ ■ ■

I looked at Jamie and just thought, "Oh, gosh!" He definitely reminds me of Ken—Barbie and Ken. I think that was my first impression, just that he was a good-looking guy.

—Trista Rehn (the Bachelorette herself)

■ ■ ■

If I had planted a flag on that spot, it would have contained the names of the only people in my life who would understand this victory: my parents, siblings, and a few close friends. Until that moment, I had been too ashamed to tell anyone else what had happened in my life. Every time I thought of coming clean, the scenario played badly in my head. "Hey, guys, I just want to tell you . . . I'm crazy. I know we've known each other since kindergarten, but now I can't come visit you because I'll start hyperventilating and sweating and have to run out of the room. Also, sometimes it feels like drills are piercing my skull, and I'm fairly certain I'm going to wind up in a nuthouse."

No, it just didn't flow naturally in the conversation.

Besides, given my penchant for practical jokes, they'd probably think I was only kidding, anyway. I wasn't exactly the kind of kid you would have pegged as a future hermit.

My mom tells me that I was great with strangers, even as a toddler. She says I used to love to charm her friends when they came to visit, and that I'd always approach them and ask if I could get them anything to drink. I didn't cry when the babysitter showed up, I didn't have any trouble with my first day of school, and I made friends easily.

■ ■ ■

It is unusual for someone with no history of shyness or anxiety around people to develop social anxiety disorder. Typically, people I have worked with who have social anxiety were shy, somewhat inhibited people all along. But there are exceptions. I think there are three ingredients in the development of an anxiety disorder, and sometimes people have the first two, which are the biological sensitivity or the temperament, and secondly, the personality traits that predispose people to anxiety, but they may not have any symptoms of the third ingredient, which is stress. So, Jamie's anxiety disorder may have been just below the surface, and then something happened where his stress level went up. We'll call it stress overload. That's when he became symptomatic.

—Paul Foxman, Ph.D.

■ ■ ■

My family was close. I wanted to be just like my oldest brother, Bill, who was popular and athletic and humble. He and I played sports together almost every day. When I was playing, nothing else existed. I didn't know about fear or doubt or all of the problems that come with growing up.

We played tackle football in the snow, baseball in the summer, and basketball in every element. We challenged each other with hard ground balls, one after the other, until someone missed and lost. Bill usually let me win, until I got older and became a worthy opponent. After our backyard battles on the basketball court, I often went inside bloody from competition, but smiling, thankful to have such a great person to compete against. We shot baskets in our front yard in the dead of brutal Chicago winters until our hands were frozen and numb.

Sports and my youth are irrevocably entwined. I can still feel the sweat and pain and pride of competition. I smell the fresh cut green grass of the baseball field we played on and the leather as I pressed my glove to my nose, smacking it with my fist in anticipation of making the perfect play.

In Little League, I played shortstop, running up the gap, diving for a hard-hit ground ball, snagging it with my glove—my most prized possession—then springing to my feet in a cloud of dust and sunshine, zinging the ball sidearm to first base for the out. For that one perfect moment, I was Ozzie Smith of the St. Louis Cardinals, the best shortstop ever to play the game. All my hours of practice and imagination came to fruition and I reveled in the fact that I had impressed my brother Bill, watching from the bleachers.

John was three years older than me and we had a typically antagonistic brotherly relationship, often fist-fighting and creating havoc with my parents. They were always on watch and refereed our relationship as if a Mike Tyson Pay-per-View fight were about to begin.

Growing up with three older brothers made my younger sister, Mara, learn how to fend for herself and swing a baseball bat like nobody's business. I also manipulated her into helping me practice my jump shot. "To be a good basketball player, you should learn how to rebound and pass," I told her. As my basketball went through the net, or clanked wildly off the rim, my sister was there to chase it down for me. Mara wound up being a heck of a softball player in high school, and she played on the varsity volleyball team for three years.

My dad wasn't the type to hug or say that he loved you. He loved in outbursts, in fixing things that were broken, in waking at 4 a.m. every day to don a hard hat and work boots in the frigid winter so I could play Little League and our family could take vacations that he couldn't. The only time I've seen my dad fall apart was when we watched the movie *Field of Dreams*.

When my dad was just 16, his father was shot down in the line of duty as a Chicago cop. In *Field of Dreams*, a man named Ray builds a baseball field because he hears a voice that says, "If you build it, he will come." Soon, Shoeless Joe and other baseball legends gone by come out to play on this fantasy field, but Ray still doesn't understand why he was called to do this. Then his father—who died when Ray was just a teen—comes onto the field. The last time Ray saw his father, his dad asked him if he wanted to have a catch, and a bitter Ray said no and left home. Now, on this field, Ray has the chance to turn to his father and say, "Dad, do you want to have a catch?" I have never seen my father cry so hard, not even at funerals.

My mom's dad, William Murphy, was a United States congressman. He died when I was young, but I'm told that we were very close and I'd sit and color next to him while he read the *Chicago*

Tribune and did the crossword puzzles. My mom was my confidante, advocate, and most trusted ally all rolled into one. At every game—rain, snow, or sun—I could count on seeing her face in the stands, and every time I stumbled, my mom was there to help me get back on my feet. She has always been a devoted mother and a fun-loving "people person" with lots of good friends and a deep faith in God. She looks for the good in all people and always treated her kids as friends.

■ ■ ■

As Jamie's story shows, you don't have to have a family history of trauma to develop anxiety. More important are the personality traits that characterize people with anxiety disorders: a high need for approval, a corresponding over-sensitivity to criticism, perfectionistic tendencies or at least high standards, difficulty relaxing, a predisposition to worry and to think in all-or-nothing terms. You may have difficulty setting reasonable limits—you may go too far sometimes in trying to achieve or please other people, and you may often have a strong need to be in control. That sometimes comes across as controlling the circumstances or even other people, but it's really about trying to feel in control of yourself. Children who are predisposed to anxiety tend to be well-behaved, "pleaser" types. You do not need to have all of these traits to qualify, but people who have anxiety disorders usually have a majority of them.

—Paul Foxman, Ph.D.

■ ■ ■

Joe Cheff lived a sand wedge away from me when I was just two years old, and he was my first friend. I can't think about childhood without imagining his face grinning back at me. We were together almost every day, playing sports and video games and causing inordinate amounts of mischief around the neighborhood. We'd eagerly await the arrival of the mailman by hiding out in the bushes, keeping quiet until he got close enough, and popping out with a garden hose to ambush him with water. The guy was a good sport, always laughing instead of reprimanding us. That was probably 20 years ago, and he's still my parents' mailman, and he tells me that our antics brought entertainment to his otherwise dull days.

But I think that even more than soaking the mailman, Joe's main joy in life was putting me on the brink of disaster.

His personal speedometer has always been stuck around 100 miles per hour, and his taste in toys reflected this well. Joe had an affinity for extremely fast and powerful motorized contraptions, most of which he made from the ground up. Motorcycles, three-wheelers, go-carts . . . these machines looked like products of a mad scientist, assembled from odd conglomerations of used parts, but they were fast . . . really fast. That was what mattered. (Later in life, Joe would drive an absurdly fast Mustang.)

In the snow, we'd attach a sled to the back of the three-wheeler he built and ride it around the neighborhood. Somehow, he was always the driver, and I was always the sucker who agreed to let this maniac zoom me around while I helplessly hung on for dear life on the back of a little plastic sled. He'd whiz me through an obstacle course of trees, or hang me off the curb until I almost tipped, or make increasingly sharper turns until I went flying off the sled like a rag doll. Had this been on tape, *Real TV* producers would have picked it up, saying, "You've got to see this. You won't believe your eyes."

If we are given nine lives, I used all of them on that damn sled, but I loved it. I loved the speed, danger, and the effort to control the virtually uncontrollable. Our friendship was built on this thrill ride. Being on the verge of panic was a natural high for me then, and I couldn't imagine ever dreading that heart-pounding adrenaline rush. It was what I lived for!

My formative years were centered around friends and sports, and generally learning how to become a wiseguy. Everything I did had one ultimate goal: to get my heart pumping. I thrived on competition and thrills, and probably had a double-dose of self-confidence. Except when it came to schoolwork, that is.

I went to a private Catholic grade school, where my friends and I were dubbed the "Irish Mafia" by one of the priests. In our red corduroy shirts and navy blue pants (the school uniform), we were a bunch of clean-cut kids who liked to test our boundaries and see what we could get away with. Informally, I was the co-ringleader of this group and the one who volunteered first for all our crazy stunts.

Most of the teachers there were amused by us, even if they wouldn't admit it while we were goofing around, but they definitely didn't see me as having any academic potential. One teacher whom I failed to charm told me every day, "You don't have a brain." She got pleasure from putting me down, and let me know in no uncertain terms that I belonged at the bottom of the heap.

■ ■ ■

> This kind of put-down is the worst thing about our culture and leads to an immense amount of suffering. It is a form of assault against a victim who is unable to fight back.
>
> —Bob Rich, Ph.D.

■ ■ ■

When I took a test to try to move up from the lowest-level reading group, she deducted 30 points because I forgot to put my name on top of the test. Thirty points. Thus, she was able to flunk me and keep me behind, when the truth was that I had passed that test with ease. I was treated to that teacher for two years before I got to junior high school.

By that time, the message had sunk in well: I was stupid. And since there was clearly no hope that I would ever amount to anything scholastically, there was no reason for me to bother putting in effort. Mastering the fine art of cutting class came easy to me, and I had no problem ditching the books in favor of the baseball field or basketball court.

My mother had me tested for learning disabilities, but I didn't have any. There was no good reason for my dumbness, unless you count the fact that I never carried a book or paid attention in class. So, instead, my friends and I focused on the things that mattered, like snowballing cars and purposely waiting for the police to show up so we could get into a good chase on foot. Now that was a rush.

When I was first diagnosed with social anxiety disorder, I thought, "No way. Not me!" Anxiety disorders were for shy people, people who were weird and afraid of their own shadows. People who had tortured childhoods and no friends. Not people who grew up on the back of a sled racing headlong toward a tree and challenging kids twice their size to wrestling matches just for the fun of it.

■ ■ ■

Anxiety disorders are the most common problem in children and adolescents. The surgeon general's report estimates that 13 percent of children and adolescents suffer from an anxiety disorder—that is one in eight children. Parents must encourage kids at home and reinforce independent, proactive, and brave behavior. They should reinforce when kids do things that are difficult for them. Self-confidence builds by kids slowly doing things that have been difficult for them and seeing that they will have some success. For example, we had one girl with social anxiety go around school and talk to school personnel and a few peers. She went home feeling so good about herself that she was able to achieve this goal. It also helps to have kids do things that help them feel efficacious or build self-efficacy like joining a club they are interested in, joining a sport they have always wanted to try, taking a photography course, and so on.

—Carrie Masia-Warner, Ph.D.

■ ■ ■

I remembered myself as an unflappable kid, until my mom told me a story.

When I was 10 years old, the best pitcher in Little League, I was on the hill with the championship on the line. The coach on the opposing team—a grown man, mind you—was heckling me, trying to get under my skin. The other team got a few hits and this man's banter escalated with each one, with each run scored on me. I lost my composure and started to cry, so distraught and humiliated that I could barely get the ball to home plate anymore.

As she told the story, I remembered my mom rushing out of the stands and onto the field, saying in my ear, "You are a 10-year-old boy and you are better than that man. Don't listen to him. You are the bravest kid I have ever known. Take three deep breaths, say a 'Hail Mary,' and show that man what you are made of."

I took the breaths, wiped the tears from my eyes, and I struck out the next nine batters to win the game.

If only that was all it took to win my battle with anxiety.

What I've come to realize is that I always had an overwhelming need to be liked and accepted. I built my self-esteem on the unsteady tower of others' approval, and when the panic hit, the tower collapsed. I thought that if people knew who I really was, no one would like me.

■ ■ ■

Social phobia, also called social anxiety disorder, involves overwhelming anxiety and excessive self-consciousness in everyday social situations. People with social phobia have a persistent, intense, and chronic fear of being watched and judged by others and being embarrassed or humiliated by their own actions. Their fear may be so severe that it interferes with work or school, and other ordinary activities. While many people with social phobia recognize that their fear of being around people may be excessive or unreasonable, they are unable to overcome it. They often worry for days or weeks in advance of a dreaded situation.

Social phobia can be limited to only one type of situation—such as a fear of speaking in formal or informal situations, or eating, drinking, or writing in front of others—or, in its most severe form, may be so broad that a person experiences symptoms almost any time they are around other people. Social phobia can be very debilitating—it may even keep people from going to work or school on some days. Many people with this illness have a hard time making and keeping friends.

Physical symptoms often accompany the intense anxiety of social phobia and include blushing, profuse sweating, trembling, nausea, and difficulty talking. If you suffer from social phobia, you may be painfully embarrassed by these symptoms and feel as though all eyes are focused on you. You may be afraid of being with people other than your family.

People with social phobia are aware that their feelings are irrational. Even if they manage to confront what they fear, they usually feel very anxious beforehand and are intensely uncomfortable throughout. Afterward, the unpleasant feelings may linger, as they worry about how they may have been judged or what others may have thought or observed about them.

Social phobia affects about 5.3 million adult Americans. Women and men are equally likely to develop social phobia.

The disorder usually begins in childhood or early adolescence, and there is some evidence that genetic factors are involved. Social phobia often co-occurs with other anxiety disorders or depression. Substance abuse or dependence may develop in individuals who attempt to "self-medicate" their social phobia by drinking or using drugs. Social phobia can be treated successfully with carefully targeted psychotherapy or medications.

—From The National Institute of Mental Health

■ ▪ ■

But in the end, how different was that first appearance on television from my championship Little League game? Deep breaths. Knocking the heckler (who then existed solely in my mind) off his peak. Learning how to give myself my own pep talk. Feeling all eyes on me, facing the brink of cracking under pressure, and then working through it until I hit my stride and claimed my victory.

It was a hard-earned lesson, and one that didn't come quickly or steadily. First, my world was going to have to fall apart. Then I was going to have to find the strength to rebuild it, brick by brick, on firmer foundation.

And somewhere in between I was going to have to convince myself that death wasn't a better solution.

⋅⋅ 2 ⋅⋅

Lunch Money

People tend to become what they think about themselves.
—WILLIAM JAMES

I never brought lunch money to high school. Who needed it? Every day, my table of friends would pitch in for a total of five bucks for me to do an outlandish stunt they devised.

It often involved spontaneous serenades. They'd pick a girl at random and dare me to get on top of her table, dance, and sing to her for an allotted period of time. Sometimes I'd just have to sing to the whole cafeteria. If I didn't do it for at least three minutes, I wouldn't get the grub. In essence, I was a poorly paid comic.

I remember walking toward a crowded table of girls, and without the slightest tremor of fear, climbing aboard and yelping out "Losing My Religion" by R.E.M., doing Michael Stipe and myself a grave injustice. Fortunately, the girls laughed. But as I look back on this today, knowing what I know now, I hope I didn't embarrass them, especially when I sang to only one girl, possibly putting her on display and humiliating her in front of hundreds of peers.

Other times, I'd earn my lunch by sneaking behind the counter with the cooks and serving my fellow students, or by letting all my friends pile their dirty dishes on my tray and attempting to make it the 40 yards across the room to the cleaning station without breaking anything. The dishes were piled up to my chin, so I couldn't even see my feet while I ambled across the room, dishes teetering and tottering and inevitably crashing to the ground, echoing like thunder throughout the room. I got pretty used to hearing the words, "Go to the dean's office—*now!*"

These displays weren't limited to the cafeteria, though. In my window seat at the back of my history classroom, I spent my time daydreaming about baseball and girls and parties and the next stunt I'd pull. Mr. Bunder was absurdly dry and a month away from retirement. He was that teacher who wore the same outfit every day—a dark plaid 1970s shirt, brown pants, goofy old shoes, and a turquoise charm necklace. I saw no need to listen to history lessons, much less to history lessons from a man who looked like the Quaker Oats guy, albeit with long gray hair all the way down his back. I was getting an F. Which was fair.

The lectures seemed endless and never involved class participation. His persistence was impressive; he was just going to talk, and he didn't care if people listened to what he had to say or not. When he wasn't lecturing, he was showing a black-and-white historical movie. If you have the attention span of a monkey, it can get difficult to sit still through one of these, and one day, I couldn't take it anymore.

We were in the middle of a movie about ancient artifacts left behind by the Mayan Indians when I turned to my buddies and whispered, "How about 15 bucks if I walk across the room and turn off the VCR, staring at Bunder all the way back to my seat?" Yep, they were game.

So that's exactly what I did. I stood up slowly, walked from the back of the room to the front, stuck my index finger out for emphasis, and killed the power. A loud hissing noise resonated through the room. Mr. Bunder stared at me in disbelief, and I challenged his gaze, boy to man, as I took the victory lap back to my seat.

"Boy, what in the hell do you think you're doing?" he asked.

Trying to respond would have been futile. My buddies and I spent the next 30 minutes in fits of uncontrollable laughter, heads buried in our arms. Amazingly, Mr. Bunder never confronted me about that situation again. I later learned that he had been somewhat of a rebel in his own school years, scheduling walkouts and rallies.

▪ ▪ ▪

You have to ask the question, "Why would anyone go to such lengths to attract attention, and to have people laugh and get on people's good sides? Where does that come from?" Perhaps Jamie was compensating in his behavior for a more underlying insecurity and low self-esteem. For many, many people who have anxiety disorders—particularly agoraphobia and panic disorder—people would be surprised to find out that they have problems with anxiety because they seem so "together" and in control. They seem to be comfortable, but there's a disconnection between the public self and the private self.

—Paul Foxman, Ph.D.

▪ ▪ ▪

The dean of my high school kept a close eye on me, and I'm sure he never would have imagined that just two years after we parted ways, I'd be afraid to be seen in public. No, he knew me as the kid who set up garbage cans like bowling pins and barreled down the hall at top speed to knock them over with his head. The kid who gave speeches with toilet paper hanging out the back of his pants.

I may have spent more time in the hallways than in classrooms, making excuses that I had to go to the bathroom and instead roaming the halls in search of friends to mess with in class. Encouraged by friends who would egg me on, I grew more outrageous and fearless in my stunts.

One day, I found a teenage prankster's nirvana. I spotted four or five friends through a biology classroom window, and there was a substitute teacher in front of the room. Perfection! Did you ever see the movie *Spies Like Us*? I was about to replicate my favorite scene.

Sitting down like I belonged in the classroom, I reveled in the knowledge that the sub would never know the difference. He passed out test forms, and about 15 minutes into the exam, I arose and yelled at the top of my lungs, "The pressure, I can't take the pressure!" This was my best Chevy Chase impression. Mustering all the "nervous breakdown" energy I could, I stumbled around the room, grabbing my hair until it was completely disheveled. Time to free the books! I grabbed my friends' textbooks and tossed them out the window, then pointed at the teacher, screaming, "I'm leaving and *you* can't stop me!"

I think I escorted myself straight to the dean's office. It was worth it. Being the center of attention was one of my greatest joys, and with each of these stunts, I felt I had gained more respect from my peers.

■ ■ ■

Compared to Jamie, who made huge efforts to be the center of attention and acted out often, teenagers with social anxiety more commonly try to avoid attention. They are usually compliant with teachers' and others' requests and rules. Teenagers with social anxiety are typically embarrassed to walk into class late because they do not like to have everyone look at them. Teenagers with social anxiety disorder are hesitant, passive, and uncomfortable when in the spotlight; they avoid initiating conversations, performing in front of others, inviting friends to get together, going to parties, talking on the telephone, and ordering food in restaurants. They tend to have a smaller group of friends and are most comfortable with very familiar people. They can appear isolated or on the fringes of the group. They may sit alone in the cafeteria or hang back from the group at team meetings. They have difficulty with public speaking, speaking out in class, or reading aloud. The avoidance of these situations interferes with the quality of youngsters' lives, such as their ability to socialize with peers or initiate new relationships.

—Carrie Masia-Warner, Ph.D.

◾ ◼ ◾

The dean's secretary, however, treated me with utter disdain as she ushered me to my impending doom.

"You know, I think some of the stuff you do is harmless and funny," Dean Lawson started, "but you're taking things too far. When is it going to end? At some point, for your own good, I hope you get sick of being the clown. You're going to make your choices. I hope you choose wisely. I know you will. Now get out of here."

Phew! Home free. But then . . .

"Oh, and how much did you make for that stunt?" he asked.

Five bucks. That was the truth, but I had to justify the act to him. So I said 50 bucks. That way he would understand . . . right?

"I don't allow that kind of crap to go on here," he said. "I want that $50 to go toward a school charity."

My bluff had been called. And I ended up losing money on the deal—so much for making money as a comedian.

The dean's words made an impression, but they didn't squelch me. I had too much riding on my reputation. If I quit putting on these shows, if I let people down when they wondered what I was going to do next, what would I have left? I worked hard at creating that image, letting myself be the butt of jokes and letting people think I was an idiot because the reward was great: acceptance.

But when I wasn't "performing," a few cracks in my facade surfaced. One of my friends noted that I never looked anyone in the eye. And I had trouble asking girls on dates; I'd go to dances and get to watch the girl I had a crush on dance with the guy who actually had the self-confidence to ask her. Friends told me that girls were interested in me, but I had trouble believing them.

Even in sports, I lacked confidence. In junior high school, I had been the point guard of my basketball team and was responsible for most of our wins. But for reasons I may never know, one day the coach just stopped playing me unless the team was losing terribly and they really needed me. My self-image as an athlete eroded with every minute I spent on the sidelines.

In high school, I started on the "B" team in basketball, which was for second-tier players. My new coach soon moved me up to varsity, though, and often told me that I had great potential. I wanted to believe him, but I remember not wanting the ball at the end of basketball games because I was scared to make a mistake and fail. One time, I had choked when the game was on the line, and after that, I was petrified of letting the team down again. What if we lost another game because of me?

When I would miss a shot on the basketball court, I'd say, "I suck." If I made a few successful shots, I'd say something like, "Well, that was lucky. I'm due to screw up any minute." My friend Brian Musso, who has an amazingly rational and positive mindset, would punch me on the arm. "Every time you say that, I'm going to hit you," he said. His "beatings" on me made me aware of how often I beat up on myself.

■ ■ ■

When parents hear their children talking negatively about themselves, they can discuss the children's feelings about themselves and help them be more objective and take a more rational view of themselves by pointing out their accomplishments and achievements and abilities. Point out that everybody has strengths and weaknesses. If you have areas where you are not as strong, you don't have aptitude, that doesn't mean that you are stupid. There are many different kinds of intelligence: mathematical, spatial, musical, kinesthetic, and so forth.

I'd also want to know where it came from. If the negative talk came out of the blue, it might be reflecting something that happened—for example, Jamie had this bad experience with the teacher who told him he was stupid, and he may have internalized that.

—Paul Foxman, Ph.D.

■ ■ ■

The truth is that I was a good player. As the years went on, my skills kept improving, though my confidence never quite caught up. I loved the game and dreamed of playing professionally, but knew I had a long way to get there—which made me work all the harder.

At the senior prom, I was nominated for six superlatives and won five of them—a school record. Yes, I had made an impression on my fellow students.

The titles included "class clown," "most gullible," and "class klutz." That was me. I was a classy guy.

Yet, even though they fit the image I set out to portray, there was something a little painful about those "honors." My self-respect had eroded as I let myself become a human joke. I knew I had more to offer than just a laugh, but couldn't figure out how to prove that without putting my likability in jeopardy. How could I disappoint the people who were waiting to see if I'd moon everybody at graduation?

I wasn't too worried about my future, though. Going into my senior year, I was playing basketball better than I ever had, coming into my own. Coaches watched my games and were impressed with me. I had also had a terrific summer baseball season before my senior year and had high hopes of landing an athletic scholarship. So long as I could get through that last year, I figured I could go on to play college sports without worry about my academic record.

But . . .

Nine games into my senior season of basketball, I fell and broke my wrist. As the doctor put the cast on up to my elbow and told me it would stay there for the next 22 weeks, visions of acceptance letters being torn to shreds danced in my head. My safety net dissolved, and athletic scholarships vanished.

Because I wasn't able to play in games, I spent my practice time working on learning to shoot with my left hand. My friend Brian Musso and I were the first players from our high school to qualify to compete in the state three-point contest the previous year, and I was determined to have my swan song by competing again. I wasn't an active player and the rules said that all of the coaches in the conference had to agree to let me compete. Thankfully, they did. With that cast on my right hand, I made 8 of 15 shots to qualify for the state tournament.

But June crept up fast, and shooting left-handed three-pointers wouldn't be enough to secure me any kind of future. Friends were heading to prestigious Ivy League schools, and I would be left behind. Until an hour or two before the graduation ceremony, I wasn't even sure if I was going to be allowed to attend. I needed to get at least a C+ on a literature exam to pass. It was a close call.

Tossing my cap in the air on graduation day, I watched it get carried by the wind and lost in a sea of other red caps. I don't know where it landed. That somehow seemed appropriate.

And something kept echoing in my mind: "At some point, for your own good, I hope you get sick of being the clown. You're going to make your choices. I hope you choose wisely. I know you will. Now get out of here."

◾◾ 3 ◾◾

These Books Were Made for Cracking

If a man does his best, what else is there?
—GENERAL PATTON

He said he'd bring a fridge, but I had to pay him $10 a month if I wanted to put anything in it. This was to be my roommate, Abe. I didn't need any new friends though, I rationalized—I was all stocked up. I spent the last night of the summer outside with Clay, a good friend I'd known since childhood, knocking back a few beers and reminiscing all night over hilarious high school tales. The next day, I would enter a new world . . . that smelled like a big cow patty.

During the three-and-a-half-hour drive in the back seat of my parents' car, my nerves went on high alert. I was timid about being away from home for the first time, about entering the unknown. My calm appearance belied the uncertainty I felt as I tried to focus on the radio and the scenery rather than my overthinking brain. I was on my way to Dubuque, Iowa, to attend Loras College, a Catholic liberal arts school with about 1,700 enrolled students and an NCAA Division III sports program.

The campus was hilly and winding, with red brick buildings. Pretty, really, and you got used to the smell of cow dung after a couple of weeks.

I waved goodbye to my parents from my dorm window, atop a hill that overlooked the whole campus, and prayed I would find my place in this strange land. I worried excessively about what others thought of me, wanting so much to be liked and to fit in.

■ ■ ■

Negative thoughts that characterize the socially anxious individual include: "People can see I'm nervous," "People can see who I really am," "People can tell I'm not good enough," "People can see my flaws," "I'll say something stupid," "I'll make a fool of myself," "I'm not attractive enough," "I've got to be perfect," "I'm so embarrassed," and "I'm ashamed."

—Jonathan Berent, A.C.S.W.

■ ■ ■

My face erupted in a severe case of acne that first week and took about a month to clear up, which was about the same amount of time it took for my nerves to quiet down.

Thankfully, I made some great friends right away, particularly Brian Loftus, who lived three doors down from me in the all-male dorm. He introduced himself as I stood outside my door, fumbling with the lock and trying to figure out how to get the darn thing to open. Turns out he lived five minutes away from where I grew up and went to my rival high school. Our friendship was instantaneous and strong.

■ ■ ■

I had guarded Jamie in our high school basketball games. When I saw him at college, I thought, "Wow, that was that really good basketball player." I thought he would be really cocky and full of himself, but he was extremely humble. Even a little bit nervous and shy. But when he talks about putting on a show to get acceptance—that began almost immediately. He was the ultimate Jim Carey personality. And I thought his last name was pronounced "blith," not "blithe." I called him that for about two weeks. I said to him, "Do you realize that I've been mispronouncing your name for two weeks and you never corrected me?" He said, "I don't care." "Well, okay." I think that was a sign of his poor self-esteem.

—Brian Loftus (Jamie's college friend)

Loras College was to be my stepping-stone. I didn't plan to stick around long enough to graduate, just long enough to prove myself so I could transfer to a more prestigious college—preferably with a Division I sports program. And for the first time I had to get serious about my studies.

My first test was in American history. Since I had never really studied before, I wasn't sure how to approach it. The test would cover about 100 pages in the textbook, and my goal was rote memorization. I read those hundred pages about 30 times, over and over until I could just about recite all of it from memory. Something weird happened during this process. Don't tell Bunder, but I discovered that I kind of liked history. Suddenly, I realized those old black-and-white movies were about people with names and dreams and personalities.

I went into that test feeling prepared, but walked out shell-shocked. I had bombed, I was sure. My anger welled up and got taken out on the dorm hall's drinking fountain, which I punched hard. It felt like missing the winning shot in a basketball game after training for months. When I cared about something, I put a ton of pressure on myself. I had a perfectionistic thought process and a fear of failure, which I now know contributes to panic and anxiety.

A new friend saw the display and asked what was wrong. I told him about blowing the test, and he said, "Who cares? It's only a test. Let's go get some beers." He told me that I could cheat from him next time, that he got the answers from a fellow football player.

He meant well. But what I didn't tell him is that I was sick of being the dumb guy. I had tried my best and it still wasn't good enough. The failure stung and clung to me for days, as I tormented myself about whether or not I'd ever amount to anything. I didn't get those beers. Instead I shot some hoops and went back to cracking the books, feeling panicked and overwhelmed.

I trudged my way to class that Monday and found that the instructor had posted our grades outside of the room. I forced myself to look . . . and then did a double take. "Jamie Blyth . . . A." I had to follow the line with my finger to make sure I wasn't looking at the score of the person above or below me, but there was no mistake.

I had received a perfect score. The only one out of about a hundred people in the class.

Shock may be too mild a word for what I felt just then. I had never felt better about anything in my life. Not even the first time I knocked the ball into the gap for a triple in baseball. For the first time, I had succeeded scholastically. Before that, I wasn't even sure if it was possible for me to do so. Now was the time for me to find out if that grade school teacher was right, or if I had a brain after all. I told my mother on the phone that I wasn't going to play any sports that year. They were interfering with my studies. She was astounded.

Staying in on weekends to study no longer seemed so ridiculous to me. My friends would come back wasted from somewhere or another and tease me. "You planning on running for president or something?" they'd ask. I didn't really know how to answer them, or myself. I guess I just wanted to be taken seriously for once. The rest of my friends joined a fraternity, but I turned it down to focus on studying.

My mom bragged to all her friends about my newfound academic effort, and word spread quickly. My friends' parents and old teachers would say, "Jamie Blyth . . . a student? I don't believe it."

But how would old friends react now that the clown had become a bookworm? I was worried about their impression of me and wondered if they'd still be cool with me even if I had tarnished my laissez-faire academic attitude. Brian Musso had been a friend of mine since about the fifth grade. We hung out during basketball in high school, but not too much outside the court. He was now a star football player for Northwestern University's Wildcats Rose Bowl team, and we kept in touch through phone calls. I'd check in to ask how his season was going, and he'd check in to ask how my studies were going.

He noticed that I was making a concerted effort to become a better person, and he said, "I'm proud of you." It was the nicest compliment I've ever gotten.

Lest you think I had given up clowning for good, let me assure you that somewhere in the world is a video affectionately known as the Whiz Tape that proves otherwise. This tape, which disappeared somewhere among the multitude of students who borrowed it, was like *Jackass* before there was a *Jackass*. (My friends from this era maintain that the producers stole my idea.) This was an off-the-wall documentary of the many ways I made a fool of myself for the good of funny bones everywhere—such as trying to pay the pizza delivery guy with toilet paper instead of money.

My roommate Abe and I ended up getting along well, often talking late into the night. He was different from the sorts of people I hung around with, and my friends called him Abe Froman, the sausage king of Chicago from *Ferris Bueller's Day Off*, but I was relieved to find that Abe had a sense of humor and could tolerate even the wildest acts of debauchery my friends pulled.

But I kept my eyes on the prize and learned how to work even more intensely than I played. I became Jamie, the Studying Machine and Part-Time Prankster.

My nerves awoke the most when I had to give speeches in class, which was pretty frequent. But I prepared well and got A's on all of them. When I looked back later, the nervousness I felt before those speeches became a measuring stick. That nervousness was "normal." The panic attacks weren't.

But there were no coming attractions during this time that would let me know what was around the corner. I was at a high point in my life, achieving my goals, making friends, having fun, and showing myself that I was smarter than I had thought. People who didn't respect me in high school did now, and that felt good.

At the end of that school year, I let my hair grow down to my shoulders, Kurt Cobain–style, wild and free. It matched how I felt: confident and happy being me. That feeling peaked over the summer.

After that year at Loras, I felt transformed—alive with passion, possibility, and belief. On a *Seinfeld* episode, George Costanza had coined his upcoming summer as "The Summer of George!" He felt planets aligning. Great things were upon his horizon for a change. That was how I felt: this was going to be The Summer of Jamie.

The prestigious Miami University of Ohio had accepted me, and I didn't even feel the need to visit—I was ecstatic and couldn't believe my good fortune. Confidence changes everything. I spent the summer savoring my academic success, working, hanging out with friends, playing hoops, and going to beach parties . . . and then came Quincy.

My buddy Mike wanted to set me up with a girl he knew, and on a Saturday afternoon in June he threw a party where I was supposed to approach her. But just as I was about to, the most beautiful girl in the history of the planet appeared out of the corner of my eye. We locked eyes for a few seconds and she flashed me a Julia Roberts smile.

"Who's *that* girl?" I asked Mike. But he didn't know either.

Apparently my confidence hadn't yet translated to approaching women, because it took me all day to muster up the courage to talk to her. About 5 foot 10, with a supermodel's body, the woman had long, shiny brown hair, soft brown eyes, and a golden tan. She was striking and poised and had a kind face. Finally, I walked across the yard in her direction and we locked eyes again. And I froze like a deer in the headlights.

Turning on my heel, I made my way back to my spying buddy.

"What the heck are you doing? Go talk to her! Don't be a wimp," he said.

"I will," I said. "Just not yet."

Of course, I was lying to myself, just biding my time. The "perfect moment" was not going to arise, and I was not going to suddenly feel like Don Juan 10 minutes later. Almost always, I had an out-of-proportion worry-meter when it came to talking to girls. If I found the guts to do it, I would inevitably wind up obsessing about the stupid things I said. If I didn't, it was because I was too worried that I was *going* to say stupid things.

Darkness crept in, and I watched this beauty stand up and ready herself to leave. She glanced back at me, then started walking away. I would never see her again.

Feet, don't fail me now.

I caught up to her, not knowing what was going to come out of my mouth. "I just wanted to say 'hi' before you left," I said.

"I'm Quincy." She stuck out her hand and gave me a smile that could light up the world.

"And I'm Jamie."

"I know. I was a year younger than you in high school. I was actually a cheerleader for your basketball team. You must have been too cool for me."

I felt like an idiot. How could I not have known her? Was I that focused on sports that I didn't even notice the most stunning girl I'd ever laid eyes on?

"I'm sorry. I was just really into hoops, but I guess it didn't help me any." Not knowing what else to say, I stammered, "Um, all right, well . . . nice meeting you."

She looked at me and paused, waiting for me to ask her out. Instead, I walked away kicking myself. My guts had vanished at the crucial moment.

My buddies were watching and gave me a good ripping at the end of my walk of shame. "You didn't ask her out? Are you high? She looked like Cindy Crawford and you wimped out!" said Billy. "Don't worry, dude. I know one of her friends. I'll get her digits for you . . . if it's not too late!"

Luckily, it wasn't too late. We spent the summer together, romance blooming and hands interlocked, promising to keep in touch at school. I was nervous around her, but I really liked her and wondered what the future might hold for us.

One day before I left for Miami U., I felt the summer slipping through my hands, ending too soon. I stood on the beach of Lake Michigan, waves running up to my sandy feet, gazing at the falling sun over the placid water. As I watched the sun sink down below the surface of the lake, I felt as if something were ending inside of me too.

My feet were anchors in the sand, clenched tight, wishing I could stay there forever, that time would stand still and the sun would forget to set and darkness would never come. As much as I had wanted it, the truth was that I dreaded going to Miami. The Summer of Jamie had lived up to its name.

But the sun set quickly just to spite me, and I watched my perfect summer come to an end before my eyes. I knew that I would never return to this spot the same man. Something was happening to me, and I felt a strange foreshadowing of doom. As dusk settled, I felt as if I were leaving myself behind—a ghost that would forever hover somewhere over the air and slow ripples of Lake Michigan and the summer of 1994.

Fate beckoned. Going to Miami was a momentous achievement and one I had worked so hard for. So why did it feel so wrong?

∎∎ 4 ∎∎

Lightning Strikes

The marvelous richness of human experience
would lose something of rewarding joy
if there were no limitations to overcome.
The hilltop hour would not be half so wonderful
if there were no dark valleys to traverse.
—HELEN KELLER

Miami University kids looked like they'd been cut out by a machine, like one giant Polo ad. They were wealthy, aristocratic, and homogenous, and I walked in pressuring myself to measure up. Even with my wild hair and the beginnings of a beard, I still looked like a poster boy for the school, and I was determined to fit in academically as well as socially—even if they were extraordinary people who were out of my league.

I worried that I would break out in zits again, as I had at Loras. I worried about the future, about exams and friends and relationships. "What if I don't get into a fraternity?" I thought. "I'll look really stupid then. I'll be alone and go back home with my head down." I worried about not being perfect. About saying stupid things. About all the pressures that accompany change and starting over.

Cynical me. There had been no reason for worry—once again, I made friends quickly and was challenged by my classes. At the end of my first month, I felt good about my transition. "I made it. I'm one of you guys," I thought.

My forever friend, Nathan Rowe, came to visit me during the first couple of weeks and I marveled at his confidence. He could simply walk up to a girl and make conversation, which I couldn't even imagine doing, especially in a new place. Nathan tried to give me a lesson about how to approach women. I tried to emulate his gregarious nature, but it felt so unnatural. I was fine on a friend level, but I sure hoped Quincy would be interested in me again when I finished school in three years, because I wasn't sure I'd ever work up the nerve to find romance here.

Settling into a daily routine was comforting to me. I'd wake up at 7 a.m., study, go to class, have lunch with a friend, go back to class, play hoops from 5 to 7 p.m., then have dinner and study until 2 or 3 a.m.

Professor Dyker was to literature what Dick Vitale is to basketball. He taught my American Literature class with an abundance of zeal and over-the-top passion, inspiring me to think and to write and to explore the meaning of writing in relation to the world around me. He introduced me to Thoreau, Emerson, Frederick Douglas, Martin Luther King, and other writers who would shape my life for years to come.

The main difference between Loras and Miami classes was that at Loras I was out to achieve for the sake of achievement. Here, class was enlightening, fun. I anticipated going to Professor Dyker's class from the moment I awoke. We would sit in circles and share our thoughts and debate the works of these great authors, and I thrived on it.

I was 19 years old and couldn't have been happier. Life was good. Until Friday, September 29, 1994, at 10:30 a.m.

The golden fall morning spilled in through my dorm window as I read Thoreau's *Walden* for my noon lit class. I felt enlightened, blissfully aware of the promising life I was leading.

Mark Basil, an emerging friend who lived a few doors down, barged into my room and plopped himself on a chair. I always looked forward to talking to him. He was funny, intelligent, and driven—a stud headed for medical school and a life of prosperity.

"Bro, I just got you a hot date for a formal this weekend, and I mean *hot*!" he said. "She's friends with my girl and she's up for going out with your ugly mug. Can you believe it?"

Fraternity and sorority formal dances were common at Miami, and Quincy and I had agreed that it was okay to date other people. It was important for us both to get acclimated and meet people.

"Thanks, buddy. How much do I owe you?" I replied.

"Just don't mess it up and we'll call it even. What is this crap you're reading?"

"Thoreau."

"Oh, we have an intellectual on our hands. Please share some of his wisdom and philosophy on our date . . . chicks dig that. Personally, I'd rather make a boatload of dough than spend my time alone in the woods, but that's just me. Of course, what I *really* want to do is rid the world of disease for the good of mankind."

"You should win the Nobel Prize for medicine. You just seem to care."

"Well, I'll let you study. Don't you have your first four exams this week?"

"Yeah, I've been studying like a madman. I'll be ready for that blind date when this week is over," I said with a grin.

As Mark replied, I felt something shift inside me—a strange physical sensation I'd never felt before. Originating in the pit of my stomach, a perverse and terrorizing surge of fear advanced like a storm through my chest and made its way upward. Smack! My face was blasted with a sweltering heat. What was going on?

The walls felt like they were closing in around me, suffocating me, and I could barely catch my breath. My heart raced out of control, sweat formed on my forehead, and my chest tightened. The ground moved beneath me. I felt lightheaded, as if the air had been sucked out of me, as if I were levitating, hovering over my friend in a delirium of helplessness and confusion.

Voices in my head echoed, "I've lost it! I'm going to die! Get out! I need to get out or I'm going to die!"

I cut Mark off in mid-sentence, and my voice came out as an awkward bellow, like I was speaking through a megaphone: "I'm gonna miss class . . . I've gotta go." I didn't stick around for his reaction, though I'm sure he was bewildered.

A tornado swirled all around me, and I was stuck in the center of it, unable to figure out how to get out without being swept up in it and hurled away. I had exited myself and was floating around in this strange body, somebody who wasn't me. The disorientation was alarming and the terror overwhelming.

I stumbled out into the bright morning glow, buzzing inside, and just as quickly as the bizarre episode began, it stopped. It had lasted about three minutes. Just three minutes, and I was about to find that it had altered my entire world forever.

Everything returned to normal physically, and I was left utterly confused as I made my way to class. What the hell just happened to me? Was I sick? Was it going to happen again? I tried to persuade myself that it was just stress. Just a weird one-time occurrence, no big deal. I wasn't thoroughly convinced, though, and I was profoundly shaken.

Still, I got to the classroom, sat in my usual seat, and chit-chatted with fellow students until the teacher walked in and cheerfully announced that we'd begin by gathering in a circle so that each of us could read aloud a few paragraphs from *Walden*. The person whose turn it was to read had to stand in the middle of the circle. It was the sort of class I always enjoyed. But this time, as my turn approached, I could feel the tightness return to my chest. My mouth grew dry. The floor was mine and all eyes were on me, but I was suffocating, anticipating the crushing horror I had felt earlier that morning.

Somehow I staggered into the center of the circle and forced myself to start.

"Children, who play life, discern its true law and relations . . ." My heart pounded. I could feel the sweat on my forehead. Not again! *"more clearly than men, who fail to live it worthily . . ."* My voice was cracking now, and I hadn't even made it past the first sentence. I was running out of air and quickly unraveling. My unsteady legs could give out any second, and I was sure I was moments away from fainting. *"but who think that they are wiser by experience, that is, by failure."* I was going to die, right then and there! My heart would either explode or just stop.

My spot in the room had turned into an electric chair; if I didn't think of something quick, I was going to fry. So I told the class the first thing that came into my head: that my mom was sick and I had to leave. I didn't care if they believed me, I just needed to get out. I sprinted out the door, ran down the hall, and kept running until I burst into my dorm room. My roommate was out of town, thank God. I couldn't let anyone see me like this.

I locked the door, drew the blinds, and collapsed on my bed. I felt like I was living in a bad horror film.

"This can't be happening. This can't be happening to me, Jamie Blyth," I thought. "But it is. I'm cracking up. A madman. What are my friends going to think? How am I going to make it?"

All through the day, the waves of terror came and went. I was on the apex of a roller coaster, and the slightest unprovoked push sent me barreling down the steep track. Over and over, the panic returned until I knew I was having a mental breakdown and couldn't do anything but give in to my exhaustion.

■ ■ ■

Panic disorder is often triggered by life changes and stress. This may be a major change that requires adjustment, or even a number of minor changes all happening at about the same time—things such as moving to a new home or a new city, a job change, a school change, a loss (either of a friend moving away or a death of somebody close to you), getting married or engaged, getting divorced or separated, a business partnership problem, bankruptcy . . . all of these things have stress value. Sometimes even positive events are stressful, like a wanted pregnancy or a job promotion, for example. Too many good things happening all at once is still stressful because it requires a lot of energy. For Jamie, transferring to a new college was the stress factor that triggered his disorder.

—Paul Foxman, Ph.D.

■ ■ ■

When I awoke the next morning, I prayed that it had just been a nightmare. Could someone go to bed as one person and wake up as someone completely different? Maybe today would be fine. I got dressed, doubts parading across my mind with fervor. Every little sound and movement was amplified as my body remained on high alert, so I was acutely aware of the sound of Mark's door opening and closing down the hall. His footsteps taunted me as they made their way to my room, just like the day before.

I was already in a full-blown panic attack before he entered the room. I saw the doorknob turn as if in slow motion. Damn! I needed to escape again.

Paralyzing terror overtook my body and mind again; cataclysm was only seconds away. Mark walked in and I grabbed my bag and ran out, explaining that I was late for a meeting.

Instead of petering out, these attacks got more and more frequent, stealing a piece of me in their wake each time.

I was standing in line at Bruno's Pizza when I felt the electric current start up again. Like the spooky music that precedes a terrifying scene in a horror movie, my bodily symptoms warned me that something terrible was about to happen. It felt like a blaring spotlight had just been turned on, and everyone in the place could see me falling to pieces before their eyes.

I had to breathe consciously; if I didn't remind myself to inhale and exhale, I was sure my lungs would just quit and I would pass out. All of the automatic functions in my body seemed to quit working correctly at the same time. My heart sped up as if someone were chasing me, my body temperature went on fever-overdrive, my mouth stopped producing saliva until I felt I would choke, and my breath became labored and unsteady.

"Sir?" a voice called, somewhere far away and dreamlike.

"I'm dying," I thought. "My brain is deteriorating. My heart is going to give out under this strain. I'm going to black out and die right here, in front of all these people. They're all going to see me die! How humiliating!"

"Sir?" the voice came again. "Can I help you?"

My eyes darted up and I realized the voice was real and coming from the cashier. The line had moved, so a wide gap presented itself between the counter and me. I was like that idiot in traffic who quits paying attention and holds up the whole line. And just then, I could swear I heard a thousand car horns pointing out the error of my ways.

I stumbled up to the counter in a state of half-reality and tried to apologize, feeling eyes boring into my back, but my words came out as a barely audible whisper. I was desperately aware that I was panting as if I had just run five miles. I clamped down my breath as best I could, certain that everyone was looking at me and thinking, "What's with that guy?"

"I'd like . . ." I squeaked out in a strangled voice. *I'd like to be home, far away from all these eyes, tucked into my bed where no one can see me.* My quivering legs betrayed me, and I was just waiting for the room to go black. At that moment, all I could think was, "I have to get out of here!"

"Sorry. Never mind," I called out to the cashier as I pushed my way out of the line and through the front door to the crowded sidewalk of High Street. Outside, the tears welled up and I forced them back, stuck in a state of shame and disgust. What kind of man was I that I couldn't even order lunch at a pizza joint without being reduced to tears?

Although my physical symptoms were terrifying, my greater fear was that someone would see me like this. The world was a blur, but I somehow made it back to my room. Safe on home base. By the time I got there, my heart rate had returned to normal, and the only after-effect that remained was an unsteadiness. My hands, my stomach, my mind . . . everything stayed jittery and unfocused.

The worst had passed—for now. But this wasn't over. I knew it was going to happen again. I could just feel it lurking, waiting to strike again.

What in the world would I say to my new friends? Every day, I had visited their dorm rooms and gone to eat with them in the cafeteria. Over the next few days, I was conspicuously absent, so they'd come to get me instead.

Every time I heard the shuffling down the hall, the fear would rise and suffocate me. In my mind, telling the truth was not an option. I didn't tell anyone—not my new friends, not my old friends, and not my family. It was too humiliating. How do you tell people you're suddenly afraid of *everything*?

So instead, I made up excuses. "I have to study," I'd tell them. Basketball was another handy excuse. My lies may have been transparent, but I didn't feel I had any other choice but to keep telling them.

My "fight or flight" response was triggered at all the wrong times, and I knew how irrational all of this was—which only added to my shame and self-disgust. Little by little, over the next two weeks, I became a spectator of my own life, watching my resolve and self-esteem erode and my world shrink around me, embedded with limits. Danger lurked everywhere.

I had 5 to 10 attacks every day, triggered by the smallest stimuli. Someone asking, "What's up?" in the hall could set it off in an instant. Speaking in class was unthinkable. I rarely had attacks when I was alone in my room, but sometimes they'd sneak up on me when I tried to fall asleep.

"Maybe this is like the flu," I hoped. "Maybe it just hits hard, but in another few days, I'll wake up and just feel like my old self again." I waited and waited, but my old self didn't make any guest appearances.

▪ ▪ ▪

People with panic disorder have feelings of terror that strike suddenly and repeatedly with no warning. They can't predict when an attack will occur, and many develop intense anxiety between episodes, worrying when and where the next one will strike.

If you are having a panic attack, most likely your heart will pound and you may feel sweaty, weak, faint, or dizzy. Your hands may tingle or feel numb, and you might feel flushed or chilled. You may have nausea, chest pain or smothering sensations, a sense of unreality, or fear of impending doom or loss of control. You may genuinely believe you're having a heart attack or losing your mind, or on the verge of death.

Panic attacks can occur at any time, even during sleep. An attack generally peaks within 10 minutes, but some symptoms may last much longer.

Panic disorder affects about 2.4 million adult Americans and is twice as common in women as in men. It most often begins during late adolescence or early adulthood. Risk of developing panic disorder appears to be inherited. Not everyone who experiences panic attacks will develop panic disorder—for example, many people have one attack but never have another. For those who do have panic disorder, though, it's important to seek treatment. Untreated, the disorder can become very disabling."

—From The National Institute of Mental Health

■ ■ ■

I had dreams of playing college basketball, of continuing my relationship with Quincy, of teaching, maybe going into sales, being on television, but what could I do now? It was a matter of days before I was terrified of people.

Of *people*! Outgoing, class clown Jamie, whose life had revolved around his friends and family, who loved being the center of attention, now was so self-conscious and afraid that he had gone into hiding from everyone.

Seeing people took more stamina than I could muster. My energy was always focused on routes of escape and trying to appear "normal." Making conversation felt like a grand commitment. When someone approached me, I immediately began to worry about how I was going to get *out* of the conversation before the panic overtook me, which could be just a few seconds.

Classes were torturous. I lived in fear of a teacher's calling on me in my smaller classes. It was easier to slip into the background in a lecture class, but then I was more likely to run into someone I knew who would expect me to get into a conversation. My confidence had vanished, and getting "caught" in the middle of a panic attack was the worst feeling I'd ever had. It made me feel naked and ashamed, inappropriate and guilty. There was something wrong with me, after all. Something that no one could possibly understand. I was weak, a wimp. And everyone could see it. Right?

Drinking made me feel more comfortable, less inhibited. When I didn't skip classes, I had to have a few drinks in me first, even for a morning class. I couldn't date or talk to friends. I'm sure my friends felt I had turned on them. There was no explanation for why I had suddenly rejected all their invitations and avoided them at every turn.

Depression sank in heavily, and I felt stifled by powers that I couldn't control. This thing was bigger than me.

Footsteps down the hall induced panic attacks every time. I had been conditioned as if I were in one of Pavlov's experiments, and it was maddening waiting for the next tornado to pass through. Every time Mark came by, the switches in my head would blare on: "Danger! Danger! Warning!" I'd immediately make an excuse and leave, feeling horrible because I knew he must have thought I had just quit liking him all of a sudden.

■ ▪ ■

Jamie is illustrating how vigilance can make almost any problem worse. He was now focused in on the symptoms, watching for them with terror. Since a panic attack is a fear of the fear, it was, most likely, this vigilance that brought on the attacks.

—Bob Rich, Ph.D.

▪ ■ ▪

One day when I knew he and other friends would be out, I went down to the study center. Books in hand, I scanned the crowded room for a seat. I was in the middle of the room when I passed Allison, a girl who went to a formal dance with me just three days before my first panic attack. She was a nice girl. Although my thoughts were still with Quincy at the time, we likely would have become good friends. Just before I made it to a desk, Allison greeted me. "Hey, stranger! Where have you been hiding all week?"

The room went out of focus and I felt as if I had been spun around a dozen times and was doing all I could just to stay on my feet. I was stunned, and my megaphone-voice came back in the middle of this deathly silent study hall. "I've just been studying like crazy. I have a bunch of tests coming up."

I had no idea how loud I was until she said to me with a look of bewilderment, "You're talking kind of loud." I glanced around and everyone in the room was staring at me. Hello, full-blown panic attack.

■ ■ ■

First aid for Jamie would have been to take a deep, deep breath and hold it for a few seconds. Repeat as necessary. The symptoms of a panic attack are due to lowered carbon dioxide in the blood, and holding the breath helps to stabilize this.

—Bob Rich, Ph.D.

■ ■ ■

Allison grabbed me by the hand and led me to her room, telling me she had some pictures to show me. We sat on her bunk bed as she leafed through her photo album, showing me pictures of the dance we went to, then her family, friends, events. I squirmed and worked hard at appearing collected, though my face was on fire and the panic was still going strong.

"I love looking at photos," I said. I must have sounded like Frankenstein or a caveman, someone who hadn't learned the rules yet. She stared at me as if something were terribly wrong with me. I thought I saw fear in her eyes. It seemed to me that my panic made other people very uncomfortable, which only added to my self-consciousness. I couldn't take it and needed to leave. "Well, I better get back to the books. Talk to you soon."

And just like that, I was out the door like the room was on fire, hoping I'd never see her again. Now she knew what a freak I was. Dazed and humiliated, I made it back to my room, convinced she was going to tell everyone that I was nuts. This was the last straw. I'd had my last day at my old dorm.

The only way I could contemplate living was in isolation. I went to the residence office and found out that another student had just left, abandoning a single room in another dorm where I didn't know anyone—just what I wanted. There was no difference in the price of the rooms, and I could move in immediately. All I had to tell them was that I didn't get along well with my roommate and the switch was made.

For three weeks, I was like a giant boulder attached to my bed, plunging to the bottom of the ocean, to the bottom of myself. I had disappeared within those bare white asylum walls. My ghost existed only in the darkness and in the shadows, in places where I wouldn't run into anyone I knew.

It was a big college, and most of my courses were in lecture halls with more than 100 students enrolled. None of my professors took attendance, so it wasn't hard for me to stop going to class altogether. I had syllabi and books for all of my courses, so I kept studying on my own.

Shame sealed my mouth shut. No one knew about what I was going through until my mom tracked down my phone number three weeks after I moved out of the old dorm. The harder I tried to sound normal, the worse it was. My voice quaked and I stuttered mildly, unable to express myself.

"What's wrong? What's wrong, Jamie?" my mom yelled into the phone.

"I'm going crazy. I'm not going to make it . . ." My words drifted off and I fell to the ground, collapsing in a puddle of tears and pain. The onslaught was profuse, erupting from deep within, lasting a solid 10 minutes. It all became too much and I fell asleep, tucked into the corner of my room on the floor.

The sound of knocking woke me up five and a half hours later. My mom and brother Bill had driven all that time to be with me. It was at this moment that I learned what love was.

They came to rescue me from myself. I wasn't able to explain the magnitude of what I had been going through, but more than anything, I was just glad to be with them. My paper on *The Glass*

Menagerie was due the next day and I had written it, but not yet typed it. My mom convinced me to let her do it so I could hang out with Bill. We didn't speak much about my horror, but we didn't need to. We just shot hoops for a while and let me pretend that everything was normal. I slept on the floor of their hotel room that night and wished they would never leave.

"Panic attacks," my mom told me, and I hoped that having a name for this enigma that had haunted me would make it feel somehow better. But it didn't. No matter what it was called, I was cracking up. Having a nervous breakdown. And I didn't see any light at the end of the tunnel; I didn't even see the tunnel. It was just a dungeon of darkness and torment.

■ ■ ■

My darling, funny, laughing son was sobbing hysterically on the phone. He didn't know what was wrong. I had to get to him as quickly as possible, so I headed to Ohio with the full intention of bringing Jamie home. I was out of my mind with worry. Before I left, I spoke with my best friend who said it sounded like panic attacks—something she had suffered from in her early twenties.

—Rosemary Blyth (Jamie's mom)

■ ■ ■

My mom wanted me to come home and go to school nearby, but I wasn't budging. She thought I was so strong for staying, but in truth, I was desperately afraid of having my friends see me as I was: a failure. I couldn't return and let those familiar faces see how broken I was. My weakness consumed me, and avoidance became routine.

■ ■ ■

I'm glad Jamie chose to stay in school. Often, when younger children are anxious and afraid of going to school, parents are tempted to home-school them to "save" them from the anxious situation. Obviously, if a child is totally school-refusing, you may have no choice but to provide some schooling at home, but this should absolutely be a *last resort* because this is accommodating the anxiety. The goal the entire time should be to gradually work toward getting the child to make small steps to return to school even if they just start by attending for a half-hour or one period, and then increasing from there. School refusal is most commonly associated with separation anxiety disorder, so you may first have to work on separation from the primary care-giver. School refusal can be associated with social anxiety or panic as well.

—Carrie Masia-Warner, Ph.D.

■ ■ ■

It pained my mom to leave me in the state I was in, but I insisted. She went home and wrote a letter to my literature professor, telling him what I was going through and asking him not to call on me in class and to understand if I needed to postpone tests. She must have written a convincing letter, because he was very supportive. With the other professors, I was on my own—never knowing if they'd call on me or if I'd be expected to speak in front of my classmates.

My small comfort zone was my room and the quiet library at night. I didn't deviate from it, and I took odd paths just to avoid running into anyone who might recognize me. A corner desk on the top floor of the library provided me a refuge to sit without being seen. Devoid of sound or smell, the library was an environment that invoked a feeling of nothingness and inwardness, in utter contrast to the boisterous and busy campus.

The voices on the stereo substituted for human contact. Counting Crows, Blue Rodeo, Springsteen, R.E.M., Pearl Jam . . . I'd sit in the dark and sink into the music, feeling like it was written for me.

Studying was my reprieve, and I survived the year, even earning pretty good grades. When my mom left, I had promised her I would try to make it to my classes as long as I knew no one would call on me. I kept that promise on and off, at least making it in on exam days. But I was growing further and further from the person I had once been as the constant fear of the next panic attack poisoned my soul.

"Jamie, you have to see a doctor about this," my mom told me on the phone. "You can't live like this forever."

Of course she was right, but it was hard enough for me to tell her what I was going through. How would I tell a stranger? Nonetheless, I reasoned with myself and decided it could be worth it.

My first attempt at seeking help didn't pan out. I went to the university's health center, praying I wouldn't see anyone I knew and that no one would ask me why I was there. Reluctantly, I headed to the desk, where the receptionist wordlessly handed me a form to fill out. Phew!

I described my ailments on the form, and the receptionist told me a doctor would be with me shortly. I took my seat and picked up *Rolling Stone* magazine, feeling just a little hopeful. Maybe my luck would change today. Maybe the doctor would have some answers for me. But just then, an acquaintance from high school walked by. She was wearing a name tag—an employee of the health service. The panic sprang into action and catapulted me out of the room as inconspicuously as I could manage. I never went back.

There seemed to be no point in answering the phone, so I avoided it. What would I say if friends called? But on one occasion, it rang and rang until I gave in and picked it up.

"Hey, buddy, what's up? I haven't talked to you in over a month!" It was Brian Loftus, who had transferred out of Loras and to the University of Iowa. I often wondered how different my life would have been if I had transferred there with him instead. Would I still have gone through the panic?

"How gorgeous are those Miami women?" he asked. "Are they all they're cracked up to be?"

"Uh, yeah. Everything is fine," I responded flatly, quietly.

He zeroed in on my lack of enthusiasm. "Dude, you been ingesting Benadryl or something? You been up studying all night?"

I gave a fake laugh and asked what he was up to. He told me he was getting ready for a date and thought he'd give me a buzz and hear my outlandish new stories. "I can't wait to hear about some of the good times you've been having," he said.

"Yeah, it's been pretty fun," I said, unable to summon the energy to sound even remotely convincing.

"Have you been sleeping all day? Did I just wake you up?"

Brian was the first friend I'd spoken to in more than a month, and I was out of it. Just the pressure of a phone call was enough to spark my anxiety, and I felt the air escape from my lungs as I tried to find the words. My voice was thready and high-pitched, dotted with stutters. I began hyperventilating and just wanted to hang up.

■ ■ ■

I was freaked out by his voice. His voice was so flat, and I couldn't believe how horrible he sounded. I was very worried for him. *Is he going to harm himself? How bad is this? Should he be alone? What should I do?*

I had to change the picture in my mind of him as the fun-loving, comedic, outgoing guy. He was going through this whole ordeal, and I had to adjust the schema and think, "How can I be a friend to him?" I felt guilty talking to him because I was having a lot of fun in Iowa. I felt guilty talking about girls and parties when he was going through such a tough time. Our friendship had to change. I went into assistance mode and tried to become a good listener and more of a shoulder for Jamie.

—Brian Loftus

■ ■ ■

Brian popped in, worried this time, "Jame, you all right, man? You sound like you've been terrorized."

I'll never forget that. He lasered into my condition in the course of a two-minute conversation. Perceptive and caring, he has an innate skill at drawing things out of people and using the right words to trigger the right emotional response. When I tried to speak again, the tears erupted from behind a dam. Collecting myself as best I could, I told him everything that had happened.

"Oh, man . . . I'm so sorry you're going through this. So, on the surface you have to project a positive attitude, like everything is fine, when inside you're in a private hell?" he asked.

Every word he said was like medicine. He told me that I wasn't alone and that I would get through this—that I could call him anytime. Then he canceled his date and spent the rest of the night on the phone with me. Not only that, but he spent the next night at the library researching panic disorder and educated me about how many millions of people had it, how treatable it was, and which were the best books to buy.

■ ■ ■

I should be studying for my geology test, but I feel I have to write. I talked to Jamie for a very long time tonight . . . He was so depressed he could barely speak above a whisper. I'm fighting back tears right now because I feel so helpless. He's my best friend, and he's been suffering from panic attacks since the fall—September 29 at 10:30 in the morning. It's a date he'll never forget. The panic attacks have been so bad that he's lost friendships, skipped class, didn't Rush, can't date, and basically can't live a normal life."

—From Brian Loftus's journal

■ ■ ■

Brian and my mom rescued me from the darkest of my torment. Although they couldn't cure me, they at least numbed the pain. They didn't judge or belittle me, and they worked together to help me survive this.

My friend Nathan called my mom one day, and she told him what was happening and asked him to come visit me. It was a huge relief to me to have a few close people in my life who cared. Even if they couldn't understand what I was going through, they were "safe" to talk to because they didn't think I was crazy, as I was sure everyone else would think if they knew what was going on inside me.

■ ■ ■

I was really kind of confused. I guess I was 19, and that's something you don't know at that age. It wasn't something I had been exposed to . . . maybe it wasn't on *Oprah* that month, I don't know. His mom said, "He's having trouble breathing," and I said, "What are you talking about?" You don't ever see a friend of yours in that light. From what I perceived, he was an athlete, charismatic, got along with pretty much everybody. I thought he was fairly comfortable with people, but inside himself, he was scared out of his pants.

—Nathan Rowe (Jamie's childhood friend)

■ ■ ■

But the weeks turned into months, and my condition was only getting worse. My life centered around suppressing my symptoms and hiding them from the outside world. I worked hard at keeping up my facade and finding new escape routes and ways to avoid people. It was all-consuming, but I got used to it.

And then came Christmas break.

■ 5 ■

Can't Go Home Again

It's always too soon to quit.

—David Tyler Scoates

It's strange when you're headed to your first childhood friend's house and it feels more like heading off to the executioner.

I was home for Christmas and I knew I couldn't avoid the Cheffs forever. I mean, we only lived a hundred yards apart, and it would be so insulting to turn them down for dinner. Half my childhood was spent in their home, and I was close with Dr. Cheff throughout high school, often talking with him about philosophy for hours at a time. He was like Yoda to me.

He'd talk about how reality causes stress. And back in high school, I didn't get it. His reality included things like bills, a high-pressure career, family responsibilities, and fixing broken furnaces, but my world didn't have those things. I didn't have acne anymore. I was a good athlete and had a lot of friends. What was there to worry about? How times had changed. My reality was more stressful than I could have imagined.

The Cheffs are an Italian family that treats people with warmth and respect and always forces a good meal on you. Boy, could they cook. So when they insisted I come over for dinner and my stories and excuses fizzled, I trudged those hundred yards slowly, knowing this was going to be different from all those other dinners. It would have been less insulting if I shaved their dog bald than if I turned down a meal from them.

I didn't notice the stars or the moon or the snow covering the earth. My mind focused on one thing: *fear*. They greeted me with hugs and kisses and kindness, taking my coat and immediately offering me cookies and coffee. I produced a big fake smile and said it was good to see them.

"You look great!" Dr. Cheff said. "Miami must be treating you well . . . but I bet they don't make pasta there like we do."

The hollow laugh came out forced. Thirty seconds down. I tried not to stare at the clock to figure out how long I'd have to make it before dinner would be over.

We sat around the table and I quickly became the center of attention. I hadn't been to a dinner table aside from my family's in months. In fact, I had quit eating in public altogether at college, always taking meals back to my room.

I found myself squirming in my chair, coughing, gasping to form words. Everyone was looking at me. They could see how crazed I felt on the inside!

"I'm not going to make it. I've gotta get the hell out of here," I thought. "There's no escape! I'm going to be here at least another hour. I can't hold up."

I was right . . . I couldn't. The panic attack came on at full force. My old friend Dr. Cheff now intimidated me. It was as if his eyes burned right into me and could see all the weakness inside. I never noticed his intense stare before; his eye contact now made me physically uncomfortable. It seemed that the more calm and poised the people around me were, the more uncomfortable I became—the contrast between them and me just added to my anxiety. Dr. Cheff was the model of composure.

"Make an excuse," I thought. "Get out of here."

"Come on, Jamie," Dr. Cheff said. "Tell us one of your good stories. What's been going on at school?"

"I just study a lot," I said.

"I've always told you this. Once you put your mind to something, there is nothing that stops you."

He was reaching out to me, trying to praise me and build me up, but I could think of nothing but how pathetic I was. The more I tried to get hold of myself, the more unraveled I became. My face went red-hot. My eyes darted spastically around the room as I tried hard to slam the brakes on my panic. Certainly, they could hear my voice shaking and cracking as words tumbled out.

■ ■ ■

When you're having a panic attack, it's best to "roll with the punch" instead of fighting it. Rolling with the punch means accepting the adrenaline flow. Nonacceptance, inherent in which is the emotion of anger, exacerbates the problem physiologically and emotionally. When a person learns the three-step dynamic of "accept . . . roll . . . breathe," the intensity of the adrenaline and energy flow diminishes.

—Jonathan Berent, A.C.S.W.

■ ■ ■

I didn't know what would come out of my mouth next, and I had already developed a stutter and slur to my speech that would last for a few years. The more self-conscious I was about how my voice sounded, the more choked up I became, and words just refused to come out naturally anymore. I had to force them out one by one, calculated, and they somehow got mangled between my throat and my mouth.

My heart shattered as I had to escape from this loving family who just wanted to see the Jamie they knew—the laughing kid on the back of Joe's sled. I just wasn't him anymore, and I didn't have the strength to pretend that I was.

I told them I wasn't feeling well and that I had to go. On the way home, I didn't even notice the bone-chilling winter air. I was scared of what I had become and how far I had fallen. Was there any way to climb back up from here? Back in my room, I disappeared in my bed, once again finding comfort in the darkness.

For the rest of the break, I told everyone I was sick. I stayed in and read books about panic attacks, which did ease my mind some. For the first time, while reading these books, I knew that someone out there understood what I was feeling.

My mom set up a meeting with a therapist. At his small office, my eyes scanned the room and found psychology books, plaques highlighting his credentials and accomplishments, pictures of a happy family. "This guy has it made," I remember thinking. "Money, stability, intelligence . . . how's he going to understand what I'm feeling?"

He sat me in a cushiony chair a few feet away from him. I was anxious, but not on the verge of an attack. I told him how my trouble started, and how I couldn't see my friend Mark anymore because he always triggered attacks. I told him that I was too scared to speak in class, go on dates, or even visit my best friend for dinner.

He told me I had *social phobia with panic attacks*. Social phobia? I just didn't like the term. It felt too weak, like it didn't sum up the extent of my suffering. I equated phobias with people who jumped up on chairs when they saw snakes and mice, not this terror and self-loathing that I felt. The word bothered me and just made me feel weaker.

My mom reaffirmed the diagnosis, though. "Well, you are afraid of people," she said. "Your panic attacks are a result of your social phobic symptoms."

"That can't be," I said. "I used to love the spotlight and being around people."

I saw the therapist one more time, but I wasn't ready to listen to him. He expected me to come back, and then to continue treatment with someone else when I got back to Miami. But I canceled my next appointment and then had to head back to school. I wasn't sure which I dreaded more: coming home and having to deal with friends' expectations, or going back and having no life at all. At least I had family around me at home; at school, all I had was my desolate room.

■ ■ ■

The two most effective forms of psychotherapy used to treat anxiety disorders are behavioral therapy and cognitive-behavioral therapy. Behavioral therapy tries to change actions through techniques such as diaphragmatic breath-ing or through gradual exposure to what is frightening. In addition to these techniques, cognitive-behavioral therapy teaches patients to understand their thinking patterns so they can react differently to the situations that cause them anxiety.

—From The National Institute of Mental Health

■ ■ ■

Quincy stopped by before I headed back to school, but I made my brother tell her I wasn't home. I couldn't imagine why she still cared; she'd called me at school, but I had never called her back after the panic started. I was too ashamed of my illness, and I definitely couldn't let her see me this way. I listened to the conversation from the stairway and heard that sweet voice transform into the voice of loss, something I had become increasingly more accustomed to.

It was the same disappointed sound I heard in Mark when I made excuses to blow him off week after week, the same sound I heard when high school friends had called to invite me to a "reunion" at Notre Dame and I told them I was busy. Twenty of them were going, and they couldn't believe I turned them down.

I overheard that Quincy was thinking of transferring to the University of Miami, and it terrified me. My brother wouldn't be there to make excuses for me. People would tell her that I had gone nuts. Would I be able to avoid her forever? I was convinced that Quincy could never accept me the way that I was.

On the last night of the break, I heard my brother John playing his guitar in the room next to me. He was a terrific player, self-taught just by listening to the radio and strumming along. The sound represented the soothing comfort of home. Even though John and I fought a lot, I still loved him and admired his talents. There wouldn't be any guitar back in Miami. I almost told him that I would miss him.

I made it back to school in a daze, feeling like a total failure, just trying to get by. Often, I'd ride my bike far off campus to a small pond that was always vacant. The idea was to fade away, to disappear, to dissolve into the vacant openness of the hazy Ohio countryside. Huddled up by a bush, on a stone, or in the woods, I'd study there like a fugitive on the run.

■ ■ ■

Panic disorder is diagnosed when a person has experienced at least two unexpected panic attacks *and* develops persistent concern or worry about having further attacks or changes his or her behavior to avoid or minimize such attacks. Whereas the number and severity of the attacks varies widely, the concern and avoidance behavior are essential features.
—Former United States Surgeon General
David Satcher, M.D., Ph.D.

■ ■ ■

The fear was my constant companion, lurking in my brain and my gut, telling me lies about the world. Telling me that everyone was judging me, that people were dangerous, that I was inferior to everyone around me. The stress caused by dreading another attack wore away at me. "I'm not cut out for this world," I thought. I would certainly be housebound or in a nuthouse before all was said and done. I was trapped in a Jackson Pollock painting, Full Fathom Five.

In the middle of the night, I'd awaken in a cold sweat, dreading the dawn, wondering if tomorrow would be the day I'd finally break completely. In my mind, it was just a matter of time until I did. One day I would be thrust into a situation I could neither handle nor escape from. And then what?

I drew the blinds and slept during the day, utterly depressed and increasingly more hopeless with each attack. I forgot how I used to interact with people and felt robotic, out of sync. Was this kind of life worth living? I wasn't so sure. I would never live a normal life, have a job, or get married. The fun-loving young man I had been was gone, and this sad new person looked like me, but was barely a shell of who I was before.

I became a mama's boy, calling her five or six times a day just to get me through. She'd reassure me and calm me down when I felt like packing it in and send me prayers and inspiring notes.

But every day felt like a rerun of the day before. Locked within my own steel doors, I didn't have the key. I thought about methods of escape all the time, and I'd be lying if I said death wasn't one of them. I often thought that it would be better to be dead than to live like this. Once you carry that kind of darkness inside of you, it doesn't leave easily. It follows you around like a shadow, a reminder of downfall and loss. I had to work hard to find reasons to get out of bed.

Panic was my shameful weakness, I thought. Why couldn't I just snap out of it? What was so wrong with me that I couldn't just grow some nerve and pull myself up by my own bootstraps? Maybe I deserved this. "I'm such a coward. Knock off this nonsense and be normal!" I told myself. But the more I yelled at myself, the more the anxiety dug its heels in and claimed its territory.

■ ■ ■

We cling to the belief that by berating ourselves, we'll transform into "social butterflies." But as you've probably learned from experience, this strategy doesn't work well. In fact, the more we yell at ourselves to "buck up," "snap out of it," or "get tough," the more anxious we become. The frightened little child inside of us doesn't respond favorably to such a mean dictator. Instead, we need to find ways to accept the anxious part of our selves, to hold that part by the hand and gently say, "You're okay."

—From *Painfully Shy* by Barbara G. Markway, Ph.D., and Gregory P. Markway, Ph.D.

■ ■ ■

Basketball became a saving grace. Winthrop Gym was only a few hundred yards from my new dorm, and I discovered I could go there at odd hours and forget about life for a while. I'd shoot for hours and hours in the dark old gym, getting lost in the rhythm of the ball thudding against the hard wood, the swishing through the net, the touch of leather on my fingertips. It was hypnotic and a sanctuary for me.

I turned into a pretty decent basketball player in that gym, alone at night. I even worked up the confidence to approach people on other courts to challenge them to play one-on-one. You weren't required to socialize when you played basketball, and I felt comfortable here.

One day, without realizing it, I challenged a kid who had been recruited for the Miami team, a top 25 basketball team in the country that year. I beat him. Born of intense suffering, my game jumped leaps and bounds that year. An assistant coach had been watching me.

"You should try out for the team," he said.

I knew I couldn't handle that. But God, that compliment felt good.

Joe Cheff came to visit me at school, and I worked as hard as I could to avoid him. My best buddy growing up had driven five and a half hours to see me, and I lied and told him I was busy studying. I just couldn't bear to tell him the truth and the guilt tore me up inside. Now not only was I worthless and crazy, but I was a terrible friend too.

I tormented myself about why I had gotten this stupid disorder. What did I do wrong in my life to deserve this? What caused it? I soul-searched every day and didn't come up with any good answers.

■ ■ ■

Most people with anxiety disorders spend a lot of time try-ing to figure out *why* their anxiety disorder happened. They'd like to pinpoint it to one specific trauma, one mis-take, one reason. But the causes of anxiety disorders are mul-tiple and very complex. While a knowledge of all this might be interesting, it's not what helps people to get better. Interventions that change thoughts, behaviors, and the physiological intensity of anxiety are what make a difference.
—Edmund J. Bourne, Ph.D.

■ ■ ■

Somehow, I made it through the year. I drove out of Miami in the bright sunshine, feeling like I'd been run over by a train. The future rapidly closed in on me, and when I think of Miami now, I see nothing but pain. I can see that kid hunched up in the corner of his room, trembling and racked with terror in isolation, and I look back with wonder at the fight that kid had in him that he hadn't known he possessed.

That summer, I hit a wall. I knew I was finished with Miami, but my life was so full of limits that I didn't know what else to do. I moved back in with my parents and took a job cutting grass for the town, which was perfect for me. It's pretty tough to have a conversa-tion with someone over the roar of a tractor engine.

I did manage to hang out with my old friends, but only if I drank . . . a lot. I was actually better in larger groups than smaller ones, and I relaxed when I could get drunk enough. Remnants of my former self peeked out. But when the booze wore off and I was sober again, I became even more lost, stuck in a downward spiral.

Alcohol wasn't good for me—I knew that much, but it was better than the way I felt otherwise. It gave me a break from the panic, but I became dependent on it; I linked any potential social strength with booze. This wasn't a long-term solution. How could I hold a job if I needed to drink to get through the day?

To a degree, I didn't care. I was waving the white flag of surrender. If a friend asked me to do anything one-on-one, I declined.

Friends would ask me what I did in school, and I would say, "I played a ton of hoops and studied a lot. No, I didn't Rush a fraternity. I don't really believe in them." I lied through my teeth. I didn't tell them how I couldn't read a sentence out of a book in class, or how I hid in my room for weeks at a time. They'd think I was crazy, a failure. Right?

I remember going to church every weekend, praying for salvation in the pew closest to the exit. You don't have to talk in church, and people mostly leave you alone with your thoughts, so I was okay there. I prayed every day and night, feeling helpless and small.

My mom convinced me to apply to more schools, and in the end, I reluctantly decided to go to the University of Illinois. It might have been easier for me to go back to Loras, where I had done well, but it would have been a step backward academically. Maintaining my image was important to me, and going to Illinois made it look like I was succeeding.

Three schools in as many years, and the dread just overtook me during those last days at home. How could I throw myself into the fire again? What if it was Miami all over? At least there I had mastered a routine of avoidance and isolation.

■ ■ ■

Many people who have been labeled as "shy" or "quiet" in high school look forward to having a chance to start over in a new school in a new place. In addition, other kids are also starting from scratch, so you automatically have that experience in common with the other students. Many beginning college students are surprised at how many people they find at school who share their interests.

Still, despite all these opportunities, for people with social anxiety disorder, starting college can feel overwhelming. Consider the size of the college and how far it is from home. It's been my experience that those with social anxiety probably fare better in a smaller environment, but there are certainly exceptions.

Some other tips for the shy/socially anxious person beginning college:

- Realize that your adjustment period may be longer than for others. Make sure to have plenty of phone cards for calling parents, siblings, and friends at home.

- Live on campus if at all possible. You'll feel more a part of things and have more opportunities to meet people.

- Consider any work-study programs the college may offer. This is a great, structured way to meet people.

- If you're naturally introverted (your batteries get recharged by being alone), be sure to schedule some quiet time every day, perhaps at the library or a bench in the park.

- Make time to exercise. It's a good mood lifter, and you might meet some people in the process.

- Commit to joining at least one extracurricular activity.

- Seek support when needed. For example, the student counseling center may offer programs such as classes on assertiveness, or you could talk with a counselor individually if you feel overwhelmed with college life. Most campuses also have religious organizations, which may offer a safe haven for meeting others.

—Barbara G. Markway, Ph.D.

■ ■ ■

Two of my best friends from high school went to the University of Illinois and asked me to room with them. They expected me to be the same wild and crazy guy they knew, and I was unable to tell them about my overwhelming fear of people . . . including them. I tried to play it cool, but felt the weight of the world on my shoulders as I agreed to move in.

My mom drove me to school, and I spent the time reminiscing about our family road trips. My dad always had to work, but the rest of us piled into the 1984 orange Chevy station wagon, rolling across the country like the Grizwolds in *National Lampoon's Summer Vacation.* We'd play those dumb traveling games that somehow seem fun when you've been driving for 16 hours straight. "My mama owns a grocery store and in it she has . . ." It was a memory game, and in the Blyth family, memory ran in short supply. It was always a quick and unspectacular game.

Mara and I would play Uno in the back of the wagon, Bill and I would argue over whether Larry Bird or Magic Johnson was a better player, and John and I would arm wrestle until it went to blows, with my mom calling out that she was going to "turn this car right around!" So we'd continue fighting quietly, out of the view of her rearview mirror.

Having a lead foot, my mom and her black driving gloves barreled from Chicago through the South like a big orange missile, spectacularly diverting tickets by praying the rosary. She'll tell you I'm making this up to be funny, but I'm telling you, that lady can drive.

All was well in my daydream—until we came to a road sign that said "University of Illinois, Next Exit."

My nervous system had already processed the message before we passed the sign. Perspiration poured down my face and my throat closed down. I rolled down the window, but still felt smothered.

My mom pulled off to the side of the road so I could get out. I leaned against the car with jelly-legs, trying to regain my balance and my composure, but the pounding in my head and heart wouldn't let me. Cars rushed by as if stuck on fast-forward, the sounds of tires and wind amplified. Too many noises. Too much pounding. No breath. No breath!

"I can't do it!" I said, bending in half with my head in my hands.

"Forget it," my mom said, putting her arm around me. "Just come home, Jamie. You don't have to do this. It's too hard for you."

I swallowed hard and shook my head. Four more miles to go.

"No," I said. "I'm going to try to push through this."

We made it those last four miles, and when I got there, I found a new bare room to lock myself into. My roommates never knew about my anxiety disorder until *The Bachelorette* aired. They just thought I was a tremendously serious student who had become pretty antisocial and moody. Later, they'd tell me it explained a lot for them.

I made it through Illinois using the same methods I had been crafting in Miami: I studied, played hoops, hid in my room, and socialized only with booze. In Spanish class, I was forced to give a 10-minute speech to graduate—worse than a death sentence. I practiced for weeks, but knew the fear would overtake me.

My roommate walked out of his room, sleepy-eyed, to find me chugging a six-pack of beer at 8 a.m. on a Tuesday morning. He was in awe. "What are you doing?"

"I'm kind of nervous about my speech . . . just trying to take the edge off," I explained.

He looked freaked out, but told me he understood because he hated giving speeches too.

That Halloween, a longtime friend called to tell me he was picking me up to go to a costume party. Of course, I didn't want to go, but I didn't think of an excuse quickly enough. The ride there wasn't bad; I didn't feel a panic attack coming on and he blasted the music loudly enough that there wasn't pressure to talk. When we did speak, it was mindless stuff. "Yes, I think Jordan is the best player ever. Larry and Magic had complete games, but nobody could take over like Jordan and win almost single-handedly."

Even so, I was aware of the dangers ahead. We crunched through red and yellow leaves amidst college kids in costumes into a packed and raging fraternity party. My friend introduced me to a girl, always an anxiety-provoking situation for me, and then actually stood there while I tried to make conversation.

That, of course, is when the panic started. I hated having him there judging me. He was polished and smooth, and I was going to look like an idiot. My throat tightened and my mind swirled while the heat jabbed my face. I was convinced I was going to faint.

■ ■ ■

Fainting involves loss of blood circulation to the brain. In a panic attack, sympathetic nervous system arousal *increases* circulation to the brain. (Only in the case of blood phobias is there a possibility of fainting.) I've not heard of anyone having a heart attack from a panic attack, either. Panic is simply the "fight or flight" response going off in the absence of a realistic danger (if there is any danger, it is a fiction created in the mind of the person who panics). Evolution designed the body to have this response for the purpose of survival. It's simply not hazardous to the heart or any other body system.

—Edmund J. Bourne, Ph.D.

■ ■ ■

The girl asked me where my costume was, and in my confusion, I didn't hear her. My friend went to a closet and returned with a ridiculous monster mask. The girl playfully asked me to put it on, so I did. Like magic, I felt my anxiety dissipate. No one could see me! My red cheeks were hidden; the beads of sweat on my forehead were now invisible.

For the first time in ages, I felt fine. Just fine. We talked for about half an hour in the middle of this crowded party under my buddy's watchful surveillance. I didn't even notice when he walked away. My voice was even and calm, and I was engaged in the conversation, actually listening to what she said and responding appropriately. Everything flowed and, amazingly, my attention was not on my symptoms, but rather, on this beautiful girl.

She took me by the hand and led me to the porch steps, where it was quiet. God, it felt so good when she took my hand. I wanted to stay and talk to her forever, there in the dark, under this mask, where I felt right for the first time since the panic began.

"Let me take this off," she said. "You must be dying from the heat."

She slid the mask down, and I waited for the panic to arise. It didn't.

"So, what do you want to do with your life when you get out of here?"

"I want to . . ."

I paused, just realizing the enormous limits my life had. I had briefly forgotten that I couldn't do the things I wanted to do. "Think of something normal," I told myself. "Don't tell her that you're headed for a madhouse and a life of solitude."

"I want to coach and teach, or go into business . . . maybe even acting."

We talked about our favorite actors and how she wanted to be a defense attorney. Then she gave me a small kiss. Her lips sent shivers up my spine and filled a void as big as the world.

I walked home suspended in a state of peace and the memory of her hands reaching out to me, guiding me out of my darkness. Lying in bed that night, listening to the constant drumming of cold rain on my windowsill, for a brief moment everything was perfect. Wishes tumbled out as I drifted off to sleep. I wished I could always have been that young man under the magic mask.

When I awoke the next day, I threw her number in the garbage, knowing that I'd never have the courage to call her. It was too much to handle. I never saw her face again, but I thought it was better to leave her with the memory of a whole man. When she looked back on that night, she wouldn't know that she had kissed someone on the brink of insanity. Maybe the night would be sealed in her memory as the perfect fantasy come true, just as it had in mine.

The next time I attempted to go on a date, about a year later, I prepared for it. I wrote out a list of questions to ask the woman, readying myself for uncomfortable silences. I thought I would have nothing to say, and lived up to my own expectations when I turned into a block of wood in her car. Everything came out monotone and I had nothing to interject into the conversation. It was impossible for me to make a real human connection while I was so focused on my own bodily symptoms and trying to hide all of my perceived defects. The drive was just 15 minutes long, but I prayed for green lights and a dark movie theater. The date just reaffirmed my lack of confidence and my conviction that I was destined to be alone.

On my graduation day, in a packed assembly hall, I listened to Diane Sawyer, host of *Good Morning America*, give an amazing talk about dreams and belief, commitment and excellence. She got a standing ovation. Everyone there was all about springing into adulthood, chasing their life's goals. I didn't have any spring left in me and I felt detached. Young men and women all around me were celebrating their promising futures, and I didn't have one.

If Jamie had found effective counseling, he could have avoided years of misery and self-torture. The longer you've been practicing a habit, the more established it gets. Emotions, moods, feelings, and thoughts can be habitual and highly automatic as a result. The best time for couples counseling is in the honeymoon stage. The best time to give up smoking is before the first cigarette. And the best time to get rid of panic attacks is before they become established as a habit. When you feed a fear, it grows. To have it die, you need to starve it. And when it is strong, that takes some doing.

—Bob Rich, Ph.D.

When I look back on photographs of that day, I see lost young eyes, a hopeless soul mired in panic. There wasn't one picture that showed a smile on my face.

"You did it! You made it! Do you even realize what an accomplishment this is, Jamie? Graduating in four years after changing schools three times?" my mom asked, tears streaming down her face.

It didn't make me feel any better. I didn't have those dreams that Diane had spoken of. My dreams had been stolen. I stumbled into the "real world" closer to death than to life.

▪▪ 6 ▪▪

Getting into the Ring

If there is no struggle, there is no progress.
—FREDERICK DOUGLASS

I had two choices: fight this thing or give up. Neither choice seemed appealing. The path I was on was dismal and barren; every day I just waited to see if today was the day I'd get carted off to the loony bin. I was convinced that I was crazy, and all the things I used to look forward to now seemed like impossible burdens. But all my strength was consumed by sheer survival. What possible strength did I have left to fight this unbeatable foe?

With headphones on, I rode my bike under the summer stars and felt numb. Pearl Jam's "Alive" came on, and I cranked it up. The words resonated with me as Eddie Vedder screamed "I'm still alive" with such anger and determination, as if he had lived the same desperation as I had and was amazed that he was still here in the flesh and blood. He had somehow clung on for dear life by his fingernails, like I was doing. The song haunted me.

I was alive. Barely. Three years of panic had left me worn out and beaten down. I didn't see any way to win this battle.

One night that summer of 1997, flipping through channels, I stopped on the movie *Chariots of Fire*, the story of young track and field athletes competing for the opportunity to represent Great Britain in the 1924 Olympics. An athlete, Harold Abrahamson, competes for a spot on the team against a Scottish runner. In several trial heats, the Scot wins.

Abrahamson complains to his girlfriend that if he can't win, he won't run.
   "If you won't run . . . you can't win," she answers.

If I was going to win back my life, I had to run. I *had* to. Not away from my fear, but toward it. Right into its core.

My days were spent reading all I could, educating myself about social anxiety disorder and panic attacks. I began a file of quotations that rang true for me, words that inspired me. When I was feeling particularly down, I would read and reread these quotations in the hope that they'd sink in one day.

All my friends were starting their careers, and I had nothing— not even the small level of comfort I'd built in college. There, as miserable as I was, I was still working toward a goal: good grades. The evidence that I hadn't wasted the past four years came in the form of my diploma. At home, I didn't have a purpose anymore. I could no longer hide behind the excuse of studying. And now that I had made it and graduated, I felt exposed to the elements—stripped bare, utterly alone, and going absolutely nowhere.

My social life was minimal, but I had a hard time saying no to people, so sometimes I would get cornered into going to a party. My entire goal was to survive these occasions with my panic going unnoticed. I constantly edited myself when I spoke, worried that I would say the wrong things—which I usually did. Words didn't come smoothly, and I was always trying to finish a sentence before I ran out of air.

■ ■ ■

In the summer of '96, my brother and I had a party and someone videotaped it. I watched it a couple of years ago with my brother. On the tape, the camera pans across the whole room; you see all the people enjoying themselves, talking—then you see Jamie sitting in the background on a couch, just fidgeting, with a really downtrodden appearance. It's like he's there, but not really there. Like he's separated from the rest of the room by an invisible wall. It was really bizarre, just the fact that he was so far in the background, because he's such a character who is always in the foreground. He was always the life of the party.

—Brian Loftus

■ ■ ■

The only place I felt comfortable was on the basketball court. There, I was bold and aggressive. In the July after graduation, I was on a team with Rich Kingston, the president of a national telecommunications company, and I had done very well in the day's games— our team finishing undefeated. I was physically exhausted and incapable of producing a panic attack when Rich came up to me and offered me a sales job. He told me to call the company's director of sales for an interview, "just as a formality."

He had assumed that my confidence on the court would translate to success in the workplace. "Little does he know," I thought, but I accepted the phone number and thanked him.

At home, I entertained the notion, arguing back and forth with myself about whether or not I could ever handle a job in sales. "Why not try? You have nothing to lose," I thought, then quickly countered it with, "What are you, nuts? You can't even talk to people."

Ambivalence might have let me stall forever had it not been for a comment a friend made when I told him I was thinking about a career in sales: "Sales?" he asked. "You need to be articulate and aggressive, a real 'people person.' I don't think that's a good idea for you."

What did he know, anyway? "I'll show him!" I thought. Sometimes I do my best when I'm challenged like this. When people tell me I can't, it gives me the motivation to show that I can. Besides, I was already at rock bottom. How could things get worse?

Self-esteem was my main problem, I decided. If I could just raise my self-esteem, I wouldn't panic. The job offer gave me something to shoot for—I knew I wasn't ready for it yet, but it gave me the impetus to switch tactics and get myself into the fight.

Maybe the problem was that I had been hoping to get better all at once, to get "fixed" just as suddenly as the panic came. But if you want to lose 30 pounds, you don't lose it overnight. You work at it, plan for it, and get it done a little at a time. This is when I started my "Panic Plan."

■ ■ ■

JAMIE'S PANIC PLAN

1. DREAM. Change begins with a dream, with a compelling vision of the future that will inspire you and throw you over the hurdles. Like Thoreau said, "If one advances confidently in the direction of his dreams, endeavors to live the life which he has imagined, he will meet with a success unexpected in common hours. If you have built castles in the air, your work need not be lost; that is where they should be. Now put the foundation under them." My dream was to beat panic and live a life free of limits.

   When adversity strikes, we learn to doubt ourselves and our dreams. We may lower our expectations about our potential—"I'll never be able to do *that*! I'm too messed up to ever go back to college/become a dentist/visit Italy/sing in public." You have to fight this impulse and instead raise your expectations. Choose to believe that anything is possible and that you will achieve what you set out to achieve. Don't be afraid to dream big just because you're feeling small. Anxiety may have stolen some of your past, but it has no contract on your future.

2. MAP THE COURSE. You can't just get in a car and drive around until you happen to run into your destination. If you're going someplace new, you need to plan ahead and map out your path. For me to achieve my dream, I knew that I would have to raise my self-esteem and face my fear head-on. How would I do this?

- *Know that you deserve success and happiness.* In his book *Success Is a Choice*, Rick Pitino's core philosophy is that you must deserve victory. You have to work your tail off, no excuses or shortcuts. Know that it is not going to be easy and it will take everything you have. The harder you work, the more you will feel like you deserve to do well, which raises your confidence and gives you an edge. Mental and physical fatigue can make cowards of us all, and the only way to combat that is by intense preparation. Pressure can become productive or detrimental, depending on how prepared you are. If you aren't prepared, pressure exposes you and causes stress. When you are prepared, you can use the challenge in a positive way to motivate you. When pressure closes in, if you don't feel like you deserve success because you haven't prepared properly, you will lose. Only you will know.

- *Raise commitment level.* Preparation and commitment lead to greatness. There are many athletes who are and were just as good as Michael Jordan, but he practiced relentlessly and prepared harder and with more passion than anybody. He treated a practice drill or scrimmage as if it were game seven of the NBA finals. You can't just prepare "sometimes." It has to be sustained effort over a long period of time.

My buddy Brian Musso's Northwestern football team had been the perennial losers of the Big Ten. Then one year they got a coach and a group of players who believed that great things could take place if they prepared and worked their butts off before the season began. During other seasons, only a few players stayed on campus over the summer to train, but that year, almost everyone stayed to train in the off-season as a team. They went on to win the Big Ten. Belief and commitment paid off!

- *Learn techniques to combat panic.* If I was going to confront my panic emotionally, physically, mentally, I needed an arsenal of tools behind me. These included relaxation techniques; flooding myself with positive, inspiring thoughts to propel me over doubt and a negative mind frame; exercising; using visualization; interrupting fearful thoughts; and writing in a journal to monitor my self-talk by crossing out negative thoughts and replacing them with positive, rational thoughts.

3. SEEK AND ACCEPT HELP. Isolating myself and trying to get better "all on my own" wasn't going to work. I needed to reach out to my close friends and family, tell them what I was working on, and accept their support when given. This meant that I had to give up my shame.

4. SET GOALS. Goals are the blueprint for our dreams. I needed to set achievable targets for incremental improvement. Goals are strength-building exercises and

should be based on effort and activity. We all have a gap from where we are to where we want to be, and goals help us to explore our limits.

- *Confront instead of avoid.* I knew that avoiding people and challenges wasn't helping me any, so I had to make specific goals to confront my fears. I challenged myself to go to a grocery store and make small talk with the cashier, for example. Then I'd make it a goal to call in a request on the radio, then to have dinner at a friend's house. I raised the bar as my self-esteem increased. This was my variation of exposure therapy, where I slowly acclimated myself to the things I feared by taking small steps and building up successes before I got to my "big" fears. If I had tried to skip through these steps and go straight to appearing on *The Bachelorette*, it would have been a disaster. Have patience with yourself. Take time building your confidence by proving to yourself that you can handle each challenge along the way.

- *Have a weekly improvement meeting.* This really proved to be beneficial. I started out by asking myself questions: What did I do well this past week? What went wrong? What do I need to do better this week? What was my attitude like? What kinds of thoughts was I thinking? What motivates me? Why am I here? What's my purpose? Which thoughts or beliefs are holding me back?

- *Repeat, repeat, repeat!* Brian Musso told me another story about his dream season at Northwestern. He said their coach, Gary Barnett, told them that they would go from being a stick shift car to an automatic. Early on, when they were trying to change and grow, they were a stick shift. Barnett said they had to "consciously hit all the pedals, shift the levers, hit the accelerator, steer. Every movement was conscious and labored. At some point, in 1995, Northwestern football turned into a smooth running automatic." My goal was to keep repeating the process until it was habitual. I learned panic, so I could unlearn it.

5. MAINTAIN A FOCAL POINT. Every day, we have a choice about what our attitude will be. My meetings really helped me to evaluate and monitor my attitude and my thoughts to make sure they were on par. It allowed me to choose the correct response. We usually get what we focus on. If we are focusing on panic and its symptoms, that's what we will get, and the reverse is true as well. Living in the past and berating ourselves for failures gone by will only ensure future misery. I had to keep my mind focused on a positive vision of my future.

    - *Face setbacks.* I had to accept that this would not be an easy fight and there would be setbacks along the way. To deal with this, I needed to maintain my belief that the fight would end positively.
    - *Keep perspective.* Laughter is important. Don't forget to have fun along the way, even if the work is serious and hard.

6. KEEP THE ENGINES TUNED. I could wage this battle only if my body and mind were ready for it, so I had to get exercise and sunshine, eat balanced meals with plenty of protein, cut out caffeine and limit sugar intake, and get adequate sleep—which is the one I struggled with the most!

■ ■ ■

■ ■ ■

There is a secret to achieving goals. To be realized they have to be concrete, specific, measurable, and realistically achievable. Too often people fail to realize this and feel like failures. For example, some may have the goal of "being wealthy." But this is not a good goal because it is not concrete, specific, or measurable. How would you know when you had achieved it? You could keep accumulating money and investments and never feel satisfied you had actually reached your goal.

Recovery from social anxiety can be a concrete, specific, measurable, and achievable goal. In general terms, recovery can be described as (1) significantly and effectively alleviating social anxiety pain; (2) significantly improving your daily functioning; and (3) effectively working toward your potential. You would supply your own particulars. The good news is that nearly 90 percent of individuals who go through cognitive-behavioral therapy can expect to alleviate their social anxiety. Others may do so through exposure therapy. Still others may do so with the help of medications.

—Signe Dayhoff, Ph.D.

■ ■ ■

Instead of studying anxiety, I began studying the opposite. I studied successful people, analyzing their lives and thoughts, reading their stories, and listening to them speak. Their fields of success weren't important to me—whether in sports, the military, acting, or writing—if they had something to teach me, I wanted to learn. I found it best to use the same method that people use in the fruit aisle at a grocery store: Instead of buying whole bushels of apples, I examined them all and selected just the ones from each barrel that I wanted. You don't have to agree with everything everyone says to glean some helpful information. I read about Rick Pitino, Vince

Lombardi, Helen Keller, Henry David Thoreau, Norman Vincent Peale. How did these "winners" do it?

Jim Carey wrote himself a post-dated check for a million dollars while he was still an unknown, wannabe actor. Coach Jim Valvano started each practice by telling his players to cut down the nets—which is what a team does after they win the national championship. Before Tiger Woods had ever played a pro tournament, he had already stated that his goal was to be the best golfer of all time.

Leaps of faith. Confidence. An unshakable belief in themselves and their abilities.

I flooded myself with positivity, taking thorough notes on uplifting passages in books. I compressed my favorites into two pages and read them daily. Every night, I would complete relaxation techniques that I'd read about. One hand on my abdomen, I would breathe in deeply and slowly for five seconds, then exhale slowly. For 10 minutes, I would say, "I am relaxed," or "Relaxing now." For the next 10 minutes, I would focus on my breathing and nothing else. Thoughts would enter, and I would dismiss them, concentrating only on the air going in and out of my lungs.

■ ■ ■

Diaphragmatic breathing (also known as abdominal breathing) can significantly help people who have panic attacks. When we are anxious, we tend to take fast, shallow breaths that can lead to hyperventilation and disorientation.

You can learn to control your breathing by practicing. Lie down on the floor and put a light book on your abdomen. Slowly breathe in and out through your nose, concentrating on making the book rise. As you become more adept at this, you can get rid of the book and work on the timing of your breaths: Take a long, slow inhale, and try to exhale for even longer. Try inhaling to a count of five, and exhaling to a count of eight.

You should practice this a few times throughout the day, and once you feel comfortable with it, try to apply this type of breathing while you're sitting or standing. Ideally, you want to teach yourself how to breathe like this all the time, so it becomes automatic. When you're feeling anxious, check your breathing. Put your hand on your abdomen and see if you're filling it with air, or if the movement of your breathing is in your upper chest. Just slowing down your breathing and taking diaphragmatic breaths can actually stop panic attacks in their tracks.

—Paul Foxman, Ph.D.

■ ■ ■

Along with the social anxiety came a feeling that I was inept in conversation. I forgot how to interact with people normally and comfortably. So how could I learn how to carry on a good conversation again? By studying the masters, of course: talk show hosts! I watched great interviewers like Charlie Rose, David Letterman, Larry King, Oprah, Jay Leno, Eric and Kathy on WTMX in Chicago, and Diane Sawyer. These people are the best at what they do strictly because they are very good at interacting with people, so I decided they were pretty good people to learn from. I studied their body language, voices, and the types of questions they asked, and worked on modeling myself after them.

Monitoring my self-talk was the next big task at hand. Most of my life, I had bombarded myself with messages about how stupid I was, how awkward and unworthy. Add that to the messages I sent myself once the panic kicked in: "You're crazy. You're worthless. You're an embarrassment. You're a failure. You're weak, screwed up, and you're never going to live a normal life."

Self-talk like this is so pervasive that it becomes ingrained, automatic. Now I was going to have to become aware each time I sent myself a negative message like this and replace it with a positive one.

On top of it, I had to forcibly change my perceptions of what other people thought of me. "No one will like you if they know who you really are," I thought. "People are uncomfortable around you, and if they see you panic, they'll think you're pathetic."

If I said one thing that I thought was stupid, it was a catastrophe and I went straight into "I'm worthless" mode. I couldn't let that one stupid comment slide. I'd go over it again and again in my mind, beating myself up with thoughts of how much of a human disaster I was and how people must have thought I was a moron.

■ ■ ■

To combat anxiety, you need to address your negative self-talk. This is often what starts and maintains your anxious feelings. You do that by disputing what your Anxiety Vulture is whispering in your ear. Every socially anxious person has one. Your vulture tells you that you cannot get through this. "You'll embarrass yourself. Others will think you're stupid or a failure. They'll reject you." You have to counter this irrationality with rationality. Using positive statements anchored in concrete instances of past success (plain old positive affirmations will not do!), you state, "I can relax and get through this. I can feel my heart rate slowing already. When I felt panicky at the mall last week, I did my breathing and got through it okay. I can do that again."
—Signe Dayhoff, Ph.D.

■ ■ ■

On some level, I knew my negative thoughts were irrational, or at least overblown. And I knew that these thoughts were destructive to my self-esteem. But I'm a stubborn person, and changing my own belief system wasn't going to be easy. There was no shortcut, and I couldn't just make those thoughts quit popping into my head. What

I could do was to become aware of them, challenge those thoughts, and choose to send myself a better message in response.

I even began writing down these thoughts so I could dissect them and rearrange them in my favor in journal entries. "I'll never be good enough" became "I'm a good person and I'm working hard every day." "People will think I'm crazy" became "I have lots of friends and family who love me and always will." I learned to pit my thoughts against a reality test: What proof was there that people thought badly of me? None. So those thoughts didn't deserve to stick around.

∎ ∎ ∎

Automatic thoughts occur so rapidly that it's hard to clarify what they are without writing them down. Writing down counterstatements to fearful self-talk helps to reinforce them more strongly than merely thinking them.

—Edmund J. Bourne, Ph.D.

∎ ∎ ∎

When I played a basketball game, I played to compete as hard as I could and to win. To overcome panic, first I had to change my mindset. I wasn't going to "win" the whole game all at once. I had to learn that just playing—just getting into that ring—*was* winning.

"Hello," I said on the phone to the sales director. "My name is Jamie Blyth, and I'm calling for a job interview."

·· 7 ··

The Runaway

Don't succumb to making excuses.
Go back to the job of making the corrections
and forming the habits that will make your goal possible.
—Vince Lombardi

My prunelike skin taunted me, telling me I was stalling. No, I didn't need to stay in the shower any longer. Yes, I was perfectly clean. But it was so warm and safe in there, and once I got out, I was going to have to actually go on this job interview that I had somehow called to set up—undoubtedly in a moment of temporary insanity. Could I tell them that? Nah, I needed a better excuse.

"My car broke down." "My dog ate my tie." No. *No!* I was going through with this thing. Definitely. Maybe.

The new suit hanging in my closet looked so out of place. I was from a blue-collar family and this was a suit from a foreign world. But I slipped into it and stood in front of the mirror. The transformation was remarkable.

I looked like Johnny Wallstreet, as if God had put me on earth to sell. Clean-cut, polished, all-American. To the outside world, I appeared confident, like I had the world in the palm of my hands.

Inside, I was busy practicing my breathing exercises and saying, "I can, I can, I can," again and again. Fake it till you make it.

Petrified, I drove to the office, contemplating at every stoplight whether or not to turn around and get back into bed. "You have nothing to lose," I reminded myself. "If you screw this up, nothing will change." Not exactly an inspiring pep talk, but it was the best I could muster at the time.

Rich greeted me with a booming smile and firm handshake. "I bet you could slam dunk in that suit," he said. I laughed sheepishly, and he introduced me to Jack Mullins, the director of sales. "This kid is an animal, Mullins. You should see him kick ass on the court. He's gonna be our top producer. Aren't you, kid?"

"I hope so," I said in a crackly voice. More nervous laughter. I was so out of my element and just counting the seconds—was I going to make it through the next 10 minutes?

Mullins led me down the hall to his office, leaving a trail of confidence and charisma in his wake. You could tell that he had done very well for himself. He looked like Gordon Gecko in the 1980s flick *Wall Street*, with slicked back hair and an attitude to match. I sat directly across from him, eyeball to eyeball, feeling hopelessly inadequate and disturbingly foreign.

"You look money," he said. "The ladies must treat you just fine. We'll have to hit the town one of these nights. You're gonna kill. I can tell." I had yet to utter a word.

Trembling inside, my thoughts shifted from "I can, I can" to "What the hell am I doing here? I'm going to bust into tears. Get me the hell out of here!" I could feel the sweat torpedoing down my armpits, seeping into my brand-new suit. The suit that made me look nothing whatsoever like I felt.

"Why do you think you're going to kick ass in sales? What are your strengths?" Mullins asked. I must have given him a blank stare, because he elaborated: "Brag to me a little. Tell me what you're made of."

"Jell-o," I thought, but managed not to say. Instead, what I said came out more like, "Um, 'cause I like people, I work hard, and, um . . . I just think I'll do okay." This was my best effort to sound confident, but it fell short. By a few thousand yards. The guy was a polished business executive, and I withered like three-day-old lettuce in his presence.

Mullins was a nice guy, but I could tell I was making him edgy with my twitchy nervousness. I stammered my way through a few similar questions before he told me the meeting was over and that he would call me in a week or so. Then he walked me out.

Back in the car, I knew I had blown it. Maybe it was for the best, anyway. I had probably just done it to prove to myself that I wouldn't back out. Going back to cutting lawns would be safe and nonconfrontational. No big deal.

Except that I got the call. I could start work that week.

That's when I ran away from home.

Oh, don't get me wrong—I know I was 22 and probably too old to be considered a runaway, but that's what I was. Opportunity knocked and I sneaked out the back door and tried to convince it I wasn't home.

I took off in the middle of the night. Suitcase in hand, I passed my brother in the stairway. He asked me where I was going and I said "New York." He thought I was kidding. I didn't tell my parents or anyone else; I just left.

Friends had always told me I was good-looking and could be a model. Now, faced with the offer to take a serious job where I'd have to talk to people every day, I decided modeling would be a far better option. After all, models don't have to talk. You just stand there and pose. I could do that.

With $5 and a checkbook, I was on my way to New York City in a dented silver Chevy Nova that friends had dubbed "the golf cart." It barely cracked 60 and basically had no brakes. The gear shifter would occasionally pop off in my hands, too. It was a disaster on wheels. Once, when the brakes had given out completely and I had somehow coasted to my parents' house, my dad angrily set out to fix the car, muttering, "Only an idiot or a moron drives a car with no brakes!"

"Dad, those are the same things—idiot, moron."

"Well, you're both of them!" he shot back.

I smiled as I thought about my dad, how much I admired him for his dirt-under-the-fingernails work ethic. The smile faded as I wondered how disappointed he would be when he realized I was chickening out of this job opportunity. Regardless, fleeing felt like my only option.

I stopped at a gas station to ask the attendant how to get to New York, and he made it sound pretty simple. Truth is, it might have been simple if not for my lack of cash.

Gas stations out of state didn't want my checks. I sweet-talked my way into paying by check in Ohio, but Pennsylvania wasn't having it. I wasn't nervous talking to these strangers; I knew I'd never see them again, so my image and reputation weren't on my mind. If they judged me badly, I'd be on my way in a minute anyway.

The gas station attendants threatened to call the police because I couldn't pay for the gas I'd used to fill up my car. I asked them to give me half an hour. I don't remember if I left some form of collateral, but they agreed to let me run to a bank to try to work some magic. When that failed, I went to a grocery store and convinced a cashier to let me write a $50 check for a sandwich. The change would fund my gas and tolls for the rest of the trip.

But once I got to New York, I found that hotels wouldn't take my checks, either. By then, I had been awake for 28 hours and in the car for 12, and the torrential downpour matched my mood. Logistics were against me when I tried to figure out where I could sleep and leave my car. When I tried to catch some sleep at a rest stop, I was awakened by half a dozen shady locals surrounding my car, circling it and staring. I got out of there as fast as I could.

It wasn't meant to be. By calling 411, I reached my uncle John, who lived on Lake George. He was shocked when I told him I wanted to come for a visit. Although he was my closest relative, I had never been to his house since he moved to New York. But he gladly gave me directions and I made it there six hours later, fighting to stay awake the whole way through thunderstorms and winding mountain roads.

Uncle John let me pour my heart out and tell him what was going on and why I was "on the run." He calmed me down and let me stick around for three weeks while I worked on my nerve. I slothed around and soaked in his tough love, knowing his advice was sound. I wanted more out of myself than to be a model. I hadn't studied and worked my tail off in school to stand in front of a camera.

"Call Rich," my uncle counseled. "Ask him if you can still have the job."

I nodded, but still had my doubts. How could I commit to something like this when I had just spent the past three years on the cusp of a nervous breakdown? The high-tech sales world was high-pressure and socially demanding. I'd have to face people one-on-one every day . . . people who wouldn't always be kind or understanding. People who might be openly hostile and critical of me.

It wouldn't be like college, where my mom could talk to my teachers and ask them not to call on me in class. It wouldn't be like a party, where I could sink into the scenery and drink myself silly. No, this was the real world, where I'd have to show up and speak and not go running out of the room five days a week. Forget it. I couldn't handle it, I told myself.

But then the cartoon characters popped up, one on each shoulder, to battle it out. One side of me said I couldn't, and the other said, "Avoiding things isn't getting you anywhere. The more you avoid, the smaller your world becomes, and the more anxious you are." My life was so desolate, and if I didn't do something to shake things up, it would always stay that way.

I returned to Chicago a determined man. It was time to confront my fear head-on, something I had yet to do. By now I had realized that I wasn't going to suddenly feel at ease with people, but I had to learn how to become comfortable feeling uncomfortable. All of the reading about success and theorizing in the world wasn't going to help until I stuck my guts on the line and learned how to acclimate myself to the fear.

Dr. Cheff wasn't a psychologist, but he was a medical doctor. I stood on his doorstep and tentatively knocked. Once inside, I told him the truth about all I had been going through and what I was trying to achieve. He prescribed Xanax for me, and I was to take it when the anxiety really flared up. At that time, the selective serotonin reuptake inhibitors like Paxil and Zoloft weren't well known for anxiety disorders. I clutched that little bottle and hoped it would hold the secret for keeping my attacks away.

"Rich," I said on the phone, a month after the interview, "Can I still take that job?"

The next day, I walked into the office on the verge of vomiting. My nerves played "Whack-a-Mole" with my internal organs, and my head spun. My legs felt frail and wobbly, and no breathing exercises could have saved me from the distinct feeling that I had just surfaced after being stuck underwater for five minutes and had to suck in all the air I could before my lungs collapsed.

Twenty other sales reps stared at me as I entered the office. They were all older than I was, and, according to my twisted mind, they were superior human beings. My first sales manager, Ken, greeted me with an easy smile. "You must be Jamie," he said.

How would you feel if somebody jumped out at you in a dark alley and stuck a gun to your head? That's about how I felt. But this was how I felt around most people, so it was nothing new. I nodded and offered up my clammy hand for the shaking.

■ ■ ■

You feel your heart racing, like you're on the brink of just losing control. It's like you've got this neon sign hovering above you saying, "I'm crazy and I'm weak!"
—Jamie on *The Oprah Winfrey Show*

■ ■ ■

For the first week, I successfully buried my head in telecom and Internet manuals. Luckily for me, this was a job necessity; the product was complex and I had a whole new language to learn. It afforded me the opportunity to keep to myself and not speak much.

The Xanax wasn't effective for me. I ended up taking it about 20 times in total, but if it offered me any help at all, it was minor. I added in valerian, kava kava, and calming teas, and just wound up exhausted . . . and still anxious. Everyone's brains are wired differently, though, which is why there are so many different drugs and herbs for anxiety. What works wonders for one person may do nothing for another.

Still, somewhere inside, I knew that if I did find a pill that helped me, I'd never really know if I had recovered. I would always credit the medicine and believe I couldn't beat this thing on my own. I didn't just want to mask the symptoms of my anxiety; I wanted to prove to myself that I could stand up to those symptoms and show them who was boss. I had to get used to the terror until it no longer had any power over me. Of course, it wasn't any fun getting there.

■ ■ ■

For panic disorder, there is a behavioral component. It's not just medication alone. It's never medication alone. I think the major strategy is to block the panic attacks before they arrive, and there are only two agents that do this quite effectively: Klonopin and Xanax. All antianxiety medications have to be tapered, because your body gets used to these medications and there is a withdrawal when you come off. But there's nothing to be afraid of about the withdrawal. All you have to do is to taper down slowly. I think the risk of anxiety disorder limiting people's performance, socialization, work, and comings and goings in their lives is much more dangerous and threatening than addiction.

The main side effect is being tired. Often, you'll get used to it in a few days. I start with low doses and then slowly build up, and usually I tell my patients they may feel a little groggy or fuzzy for a few days—it's like taking antihistamine. But after, you should ideally not know that your body is taking anything. The good thing about Xanax and Klonopin is they don't tend to be drugs of abuse because you don't get a high or a buzz off them, unlike Valium.

The other medication that has been used successfully for panic attacks is the so-called SSRIs (selective serotonin reuptake inhibitors), which are antidepressants. There is a very close link between anxiety and depression. Many people with anxiety disorders get clinical depression. SSRIs such as Prozac, Zoloft, and Paxil have been used to prevent panic attacks and treat anxiety disorders. They increase serotonin in the brain by preventing it from being reabsorbed by the cells. They are not as immediately effective—they take a while to work. The brain has to build up serotonin.

I find that starting somebody on Klonopin and helping them realize it's really going to help them prevent the panic attacks, then gradually introducing an SSRI like Prozac or Zoloft is a good method.

The antidepressants tend to have less of a withdrawal than the other medications. If someone is also both depressed and anxious, you can improve both conditions with just one medication. Antidepressants are also very helpful for other anxiety disorders like generalized anxiety disorder, social phobia, and PTSD. The SSRIs are well tolerated and have few side effects.

Those with anxiety disorders are among the hardest people to convince that medications can help them. One thing we have to understand is that anxiety disorders are biological problems. Other illnesses—for example, migraines, allergies, and gastrointestinal problems—all have significant psychological and stress-related components and yet we all agree that you take medications for these. But there is a huge unwarranted stigma about getting treatment for anxiety.

Anxiety is biological, psychological, and social, and if you don't address any one of those, you're really not giving yourself the best shot at reducing it. If somebody comes to me with an anxiety disorder, I explain to them that the psychological techniques are going to be the major part of the treatment, but I also explain that real relief can come from medication. In my view, if you do both, you get the best results.

—Eugene Beresin, M.D.

■ ■ ■

One of the more established sales reps went over a sales and product manual with me during that first week on the job. The guy was really nice and was trying to help me understand, but I grew more frayed with every page he flipped. When he quizzed me after demonstrating something, I was at a loss. Because I had been falling apart emotionally, I couldn't listen to a word. I thought, "This guy must think I'm crazy or just plain stupid." He never did the training with me again—either he realized I was too frazzled to handle it, or he just thought I was a lost cause.

Ken taught us collectively, which made me feel more at ease. This, of course, is relative—my "more at ease" was probably comparable to other people's torment. But I had grown accustomed to this constant buzzing of fraught nerves. That didn't make it easy, but it was less terrifying than those first few weeks at Miami when I had no idea what was happening to me.

Ken didn't make anybody participate during his training, so I, of course, never did. I wasn't the center of attention, and I didn't have to worry about being called on to speak. I just listened as he went over our product set, sales strategy, territories, quotas, expectations, and goals.

I accompanied him on a few sales calls the following week. He sensed that I was fragile, and although he put pressure on all of us, I felt that he was looking out for me. On these calls, I could just listen, learning the trade and art of sales, of breaking people down and making them do things they originally had no desire to do.

This was the tech boom of the late 1990s; the economy was going through the roof, and so was our company. Its stock was skyrocketing and the pressure was on for all of us to grab pieces of the pie for our nascent business. The stakes were high and the pressure was always on. Our CEO used to say that it was not a company for the faint of heart. We sold phone services, Internet access and Web site hosting, data networking products, and wireless services. Or, at least, Ken sold those things. I watched.

Then Rich called for a Chicago-wide meeting of all the sales reps at the Wyndham Garden Hotel. It was my second week on the job, and I had steeled myself only for the experience of sitting and watching lectures and presentations. Instead, he announced, he wanted each of the sales reps to go up on stage and perform a role-play with him.

"It's sales pitch time, and I'm your customer. You're going to get up here and do your best to sell me . . . and it won't be easy."

There were two chairs on center stage placed inches away from each other, face-to-face, creating an intimidating aura. One by one, I watched my colleagues give it their all, then get panned and berated by our president. I, on the other hand, thought they were great.

From my chair, the stage looked like a giant torture chamber. This was a sick game, and I felt like I was about to get my teeth ripped out of my mouth. Nobody had any idea of how scared I was, but I was about to be exposed. I was sure the people next to me could hear my heart beating. It pounded so hard that my ears throbbed.

Panic was a conditioned response, and it flooded me, escalating as my turn approached. Forget trying to pay attention and learn from the others' presentations. All I could do was to fight off my symptoms and beg for mercy.

One of the management superiors, an ex-Army ranger, sat next to me and said, "You getting ready, son? Can't wait to put you on the hot seat. See how you fare. Sales takes confidence. Let's see what you got."

My eyes brimmed with tears and I bit hard on my lip to hold back the torrent. It was so painful I could barely speak, but I told him I was scared.

"Who cares if you screw up? It's all about learning," he said.

Learning, my ass. I was sending myself to be humiliated, to break down like a little kid on display in a room full of colleagues. "You have no idea the hell I'm going through, buddy!" I thought. Nor did I want him to find out what I was going through! I was completely unglued and ready to self-destruct just looking at the chairs and the microphone underneath the bright white spotlight. The positive thinking didn't even surface. This was my opportunity to put the Panic Plan to the test, and I failed miserably.

I heard my number called and stood in a trance.

"Jamie, come on up here and show these boys how it's done!" Rich said. I was his discovery on the basketball court and now he wanted to show off his prize. I later found out that Rich had already gone to bat for me. After my shaky interview, the sales director didn't want to hire me. Rich insisted. When it came to people, Rich said he always went with his gut. And to add to the pressure, I was the first rep they'd ever hired right out of college, and now I was to be the guinea pig for all future recent college grads. If I succeeded, they'd hire more. If I failed, the door was closed. Guess which way I felt the door swinging while I forced myself out of my seat?

Two hundred men and women offered me a small, customary round of applause as I made my way to the stage. Before I even sat down in that hard folding chair, I was in the middle of a full-blown panic attack, and as my eyes involuntarily darted around the room, every face in the crowd was a blur. Even though I couldn't see them, I could feel them staring at me, burning holes through me, peering right into my weakness and seeing a madman.

My nightmare unfolded before my eyes. I wasn't prepared for this. A storm raged inside me, telling me my life was over as I tried to appear calm. The tears knotted up in my throat and my chest ached with humiliation.

I wanted to wave the white flag and run. I was cooked before I even began—breathless, voiceless, and losing my tenuous grip on reality. It was too much, and all I could think about was how to end this pain. I needed to escape, and this time, I didn't ever want to return.

I pictured a train, but I wasn't getting on it to escape; I was lying under it. The thought of being pulverized by its force brought a strange sensation of relief. No more fighting. This would be my final surrender.

As I was about to get up and run out of the room, our president got a call on his cell phone. It was an emergency from the corporate office.

"Meeting's off," he said. "We'll finish this next week."

Everybody scurried off, and my panic subsided as the room emptied. If that phone call hadn't come through, I would have broken down crying in front of 200 grown men and women. I walked out to my car that October afternoon a beaten man, feeling numb and empty. I didn't feel like crying anymore. My thoughts weren't even spiraling out of control. I was just done. I was at the end of myself.

Down at the tracks, I watched the trains barrel by, thinking about the swiftness of their force. Thinking about finality and escape. Flat pennies, flat bones, flat lives. As I sat on the hood of my car, the screaming of the train whistle mixed with the screaming pain in my heart until everything intertwined and nothing mattered anymore.

·· 8 ··

On a Mission

The gem cannot be polished without friction,
nor a man perfected without trials.
—Chinese proverb

"How did the meeting go?" my mom asked on the phone.

"Fine," I lied.

"Oh, Jamie, you did it!" she said. "Let's go out to dinner to celebrate."

I peeled myself out of my suit and into jeans, feeling like an awful fraud. Lying to my mother wasn't my style, but it was better than letting her know that her son was contemplating flattening himself under a train.

Once at the restaurant with mom and Bill, though, I couldn't keep up the ruse. They asked too many questions and I dissolved right in the middle of Bennigan's over a plate of spaghetti.

"I can't do it. I can't do it," I said, erupting into the stored-up onslaught of tears that I had held back earlier. They gushed out like a faucet and I choked on my words, sobbing like never before. My face fell into the plate of pasta. I didn't even care if anyone saw me. I couldn't stop. I had thrown myself into the fire—why was I surprised that I got burned?

There would be another meeting next week, and I was going to face this all over again. The same anticipation, the same panic, and this time, no cell phone would save me.

They tried to boost me with a pep talk, but I was inconsolable. Then my mom switched tactics.

"This is nuts. You go to that meeting, thank them for the opportunity, and come home. This is just too hard," she said.

"I feel like a failure," I said.

"Sales just isn't right for you, and that's okay," she said. "It's the effort that counts and you're brave for trying. It's okay to quit."

She says otherwise, but I think she knew just what she was doing: she was lighting a fire under me, just the same way my old roommate had done when he told me I couldn't do it. By telling me she thought I should quit, she had just laid down the gauntlet; now I had to decide if I was up for the challenge of proving her wrong.

The choice was mine, and I was at a crossroads: fight or give up. It was one of the most difficult choices I'd ever made, and it wound up being the turning point of my life. Everyone, at some point or another, comes to a defining moment where the next action will change the course of his or her life. This was mine, and I chose to fight.

I went home and wrote a mission statement: "Panic is not going to stop me. I am not going to quit."

With one week to go before the dreaded role-play, I prepared myself for the task at hand. I practiced my sales pitch day and night. Somewhere, I read about visualization and how effective it was for athletes. Several studies have been done to prove this. Australian psychologist Alan Richardson showed that students could improve their free throws in basketball by 23 percent just by spending time every day lying down and visualizing themselves making the shots—even though they didn't actually touch a basketball during the 20 days of the experiment! He said it worked best when the students used several senses—"feeling" the ball, "hearing" it bounce, and "seeing" it go through the hoop, for example.

Phil Jackson of the World Champion Chicago Bulls used to make players like Jordan, Rodman, and Pippen sit around in a circle every practice to meditate, do breathing techniques, and visualize their success. He knew this would help them relax and become more confident on the court. Our bodies' nervous systems don't know the difference between what's real and what's imagined, so a good visualization can "train" us for a situation nearly as well as physically practicing it.

■ ■ ■

I use guided imagery personally, and teach it to most of my clients. It is the most powerful device we can use: for our benefit, or our destruction. When Jamie was destroying himself, it was because of unintended imagery showing him failure. By imaging success, it could be his.

—Bob Rich, Ph.D.

■ ■ ■

If it was good enough for them, it was good enough for me. I visualized my presentation. I saw myself rising from my chair, walking to the stage with my head held high, and talking with ease. My hands were warm and dry, even breaths were automatic, and my smile was natural. I envisioned success and a good reception by my boss and coworkers. I felt the pride of success, even though I was just sitting in my dark basement with my eyes closed.

I had to create these made-up "good memories" in my mind to override the traumatic memory of cracking in the hot seat. If I panicked, I told myself, I would roll with it and remember that it was just a normal bump in the road and not the end of my life. It didn't mean I was going to die, or that I was less of a person.

No matter how real my symptoms felt, I had to remind myself of the evidence. "You have never passed out in the middle of a panic attack. You have never had a heart attack. You have always lived through these attacks, and they last only a few minutes."

I monitored my negative thoughts carefully and didn't allow them to slip by with "get out of jail free" cards. No, these thoughts were to be scrutinized, held up to the harsh light of day, and edited into rational and positive thoughts. This doesn't work overnight, but I dedicated myself to work on it until the positive thoughts became automatic.

After giving my sales pitch to the captive audience of basement boxes, tools, and workout equipment, I decided it was time to move on to a less inanimate crowd. I called upon my father, a man who was never big on touchy-feely Hallmark sentiments, but would give it to me straight and repeat this practice with me again and again into the wee hours of the night, as long as I wanted him to.

Next, I called on my mom and my brother Bill. I took notes and tried to ready myself for all possible questions and reactions. I don't think I slept more than 10 hours all week.

I went back to those positive books and quotes, memorizing the most inspiring thoughts, making them my own thoughts.

On the day of the meeting, I knew there was a cheering section at home pacing and waiting, pulling for me to succeed.

"How did you do?" my mom asked with worry as I walked through the door.

"I didn't have to do the role-play," I said. She exhaled with relief. I was saving the dramatic climax, of course. "They asked for volunteers, so I raised my hand."

My fear hadn't vanished. In fact, I was shaking with trepidation as I climbed the stairs onto the stage and sat in that chair for 45 grueling minutes, working hard to "sell" my boss on upgrading his current dial-up Internet connection to a T-1 connection.

I started with my "impact statement": "Thanks for meeting with me. The reason I'm here today is because my company has significantly improved the profitability and efficiency of many companies in the area and throughout the United States, and I'd like to determine if we could have the same impact on your business."

My voice was unsteady, but I kept going anyway. Despite the fact that I was sure people could see the sweat forming on my forehead and the heat filling my cheeks, I was not going to back down this time. Panic was not going to win.

Throughout my presentation, I had to ask the "buyer" many questions to determine his business's needs, then figure out who my competition was and how we compared, handle any objections, and close the sale.

Everyone in the room got to scrutinize these presentations, acting as if they were judges in *American Idol.* We had a few Simons in the group who liked to be brutally honest and point out flaws ("You are the worst salesman in America!"). The hardest part was that I was talking about something I really didn't know much about—telecom is very intricate. It would have been slightly more comforting to talk about the dynamics of a pick-and-roll in basketball, but no such luck. We were each graded on how well we covered all the objectives of the sales process and how compelling our case was. My grade was around a B, which, to me, felt like an A+.

Nobody knew how scared I was, and coworkers even complimented me on my presentation. Pride overcame me, and I felt a glowing happiness that couldn't be suppressed. I had done it. The panic had hit, and I had hit back . . . and won.

When my family and I went to dinner that night, it really was a celebration. I would be going back to work the next day.

Now it was time to take the confidence I'd built up for the role-playing and move it into the cruel, cruel world of cold sales calls. The job was to convince businesses to switch their phone lines and Internet connectivity to our communications firm. We canvassed the streets in search of businesses, walking into offices door-to-door—office park to office park, skyscraper to skyscraper. Believe me, we weren't exactly met with open arms.

Our objective was to get past the secretaries—the "gatekeepers," as we called them—and to the decision makers, who were usually the office managers, presidents, or CEOs. Once we found these head honchos, we were to set up a meeting at which we'd perform a presentation and write a cost proposal, ultimately trying to get them to sign an agreement. It was hard enough to get anyone to talk to us, let alone to convince them to listen and consider switching to our little-known, new company.

We had monthly quotas—sales numbers we had to reach. Every month was a race to the finish line, and from October through January I didn't make a single sale on my own. I failed and failed, but I had more possibilities in the pipeline than anyone on the sales team. Others would show up and drink coffee and relax; I was already out the door, fueled by an overabundance of panic and energy, searching for that elusive sale. I was running scared, but I was running, and that was better than standing still.

I went on about 50 to 75 cold calls a day, failing about 90 percent of the time. But every now and then I'd get lucky and the decision maker would agree to a meeting. Ken went with me on these meetings, and he was good. Out of 10 meetings, he sold 7 of them, making me the top sales rep in the office. Granted, I found the clients, but he's the one who actually made the sales, and this made the other reps a bit resentful.

Cold calling helped to desensitize me. On some days I could handle the pressure, while on others, I'd crumble under the weight, choking with panic. My emotions and performance were inconsistent, but if you charted my progress, you would have seen a gradual incline. Every day, I was forced to confront my greatest fear by giving dozens of mini-presentations a day. I even got paid to do it!

■ ■ ■

Most psychological treatments for social anxiety disorder include exposure as a component. It's not usually the whole treatment, but it's perhaps the most important part of treatment. It essentially involves getting people to confront the situations they fear, actually going into the feared situations repeatedly until they're not afraid of the situations any more. Some of it may be done live in the actual situations, and some of it may also be done with role-plays, like practicing job interviews with friends and family.

—Martin Antony, Ph.D.

■ ■ ■

Although I knew I was doing well, I had grave doubts about making it on my own. Would I be able to hack it without Ken? I was just trying to get by day by day, hour by hour, and didn't know if the extra responsibility and pressure of doing the meetings by myself would tear the thin fabric of confidence I was weaving.

■ ■ ■

There are four essential things you can do to enhance your self-confidence.

1. *Create a bushel basket full of past success instances and record them in a journal.* These are little and big things that have happened over your life to the present wherein you felt good about yourself. They could include when you did something nice for your grandmother that she really appreciated, when you did your first adult chore, learned to ride a bicycle, hit a home run, won an award for your work, had a letter published in the newspaper, got a promotion, and so on. Recall these instances in all their cinematic glory and sensory detail so you can relive the feeling when you think about them. These are the things you retrieve from memory to provide evidence to yourself that you are not inadequate or worthless and you can succeed.

2. *Record daily in your journal what you have done right and what has gone well for you.* The more aware you are of your daily successes, the more ammunition you will give your Inner Success Coach to fight and ultimately vanquish your Anxiety Vulture.

3. *Produce a list of rewards—things that you value—to give yourself when you succeed.* Like your successes, these rewards range from tiny to large. With each success you verbally pat yourself on the back, saying, "I did it. It was a success. I feel good about myself and deserve a reward." Then choose a reward that is comparable to the success in degree.

4. *Slowly begin to do the things you fear.* Prepare for them, have your abdominal breathing and positive self-talk handy, and test in baby steps your ability to control the situation and your response to it. Each success builds on the next, adding to your self-confidence. And, of course, praise and reward your efforts.

—Signe Dayhoff, Ph.D.

■ ■ ■

Ken offered me a raise, but I didn't want it. That wasn't the point. Sure, I needed money as much as anyone else, but this job wasn't about earning a new car or an entertainment center; it was about earning my own life back. Most people were there to chase money, but I was there to improve myself; if I could do that, I knew the money would follow—and that I would deserve it.

I got out there day after day and I panicked. I panicked, and I did it anyway, over and over. I talked to secretaries, I stammered in front of sharp businesspeople, and I fought off the urge to faint in offices all over the city. In the Chicago high-rise office buildings, overlooking the city through a 60-story window, I remember steeling myself against the thought that there was no escape in sight.

My alarm clock became a trigger for the panic—as soon as it went off, shivers ran down my spine because it meant I was heading off to work as a high-tech salesman. I always felt vulnerable, like this would be the day that I'd be exposed. Some days I dreaded that doomsday feeling so much that I didn't bother going to sleep at all. Instead, I'd head to the driving range at 4 a.m., when no one else was around, and just work on my putting or chipping or short wedge shots in the darkness until my mind focused more on the action than on my anxiety. By 6:30 a.m., I was already on my way to the office.

I never felt good about heading to work, but I kept going. Only with practice and preparation would I get anywhere—both with sales and with panic. Some days it was very difficult to maintain my discipline because I'd wake up feeling off and overly anxious, knowing that I was about to throw myself into an uncomfortable situation. Those were the days that maintaining my discipline mattered the most. I had to keep my mind on my positive vision of the future, not on my current reality and struggles.

■ ■ ■

If I do something brave, I *am* brave, regardless of how scared I felt. In fact, I am all the braver for having been terrified and doing it anyway.

—Bob Rich, Ph.D.

■ ■ ■

I took an "Intro to Acting" course at a local theater to overcome my stage fright. Early on, the instructor gave us a difficult task: stand center stage and do nothing. Just stand there in front of the class for five minutes. The other students were to rate how nervous we looked. As you might imagine, I hated this exercise! But I stood there and tried to remember the teacher's instructions: instead of focusing on the fact that people are looking at you and judging you, watch them instead. In other words, instead of being aware that you're the subject, make the audience the subject instead. Watch their movements; observe them.

The first time I did the exercise, the other students rated my nervousness as "minimal." The second time, they thought I was the least nervous person in the room.

Still, sales presentations were tough for me. I spoke to a friend's dad about it, and he shocked me by telling me that public speaking was his biggest fear too. This man was a successful millionaire and I thought he had all the confidence in the world. It relieved me to hear that this man, whom I greatly respected, would rather have bees swarm his head than do a sales presentation.

He told me about Toastmasters, a group that got together to practice impromptu and prepared speeches, and I went to their meetings. I was always nervous, but I never had panic attacks, and I gained insight into the way people saw me: no matter how I felt, no one ever recognized how anxious I was. This group was a big help to me.

I also went to churches and did readings in front of hundreds of people. I tried to do anything I could to move beyond my comfort zone.

Initially, my goal was not to erase panic. My goal was to become a success despite the panic. I wanted to reach my dreams and my full potential, no matter how broken I was. To do this, I knew I had to improve gradually—day by day, hour by hour, cold call by cold call, and meeting by meeting. Action fosters momentum, and I had to get my train moving in the right direction by fueling it with my own steam.

I tape recorded positive statements, and I listened to the tapes while I drove to work. I learned about progressive muscle relaxation and used it when I felt the symptoms of stress creeping into my tense shoulders and neck.

■ ■ ■

CONDITIONED RELAXATION, JACOBSON TECHNIQUE

Progressive muscular relaxation was devised by Edmund Jacobson in the 1930s and has been repeatedly improved since. It is widely used to help people with phobias, stage fright, anger management problems, examination anxiety, and chronic environmental stress. It provides a tool that can be used for the rest of your life in any situation where the "fight or flight" reaction occurs but is unwanted.

What we do is to condition muscular relaxation in the whole body to a *key action* and a *key phrase*. Once learned, doing the key action and thinking the key phrase is automatically followed by muscular relaxation and therefore control of fear, anger, or anxiety. After a couple of weeks of conscientious practice, you can achieve this in one second. You now have a lifelong skill.

Initially, you need a warm, quiet room and loose-fitting clothes. Lie on a hard surface like a carpeted floor, though a firm, comfortable armchair will do, preferably with a head-rest. If lying, use a small pillow to support your head, but not under the shoulders. Have your arms by your side, feet uncrossed. You may need a blanket to cover you, because your body temperature will fall as you relax.

Research has shown that muscles can be relaxed in 16 large groups:

> Right lower arm and hand [tighten the fist and
>   hold it; let hand go loose]
>
> Left lower arm and hand
>
> Right upper arm [without tensing or moving the
>   lower arm, bunch up the upper arm muscles

like Popeye after he's had spinach; allow lower arm to drop]

Left upper arm

Right lower leg [point your toes like a ballerina, but beware of cramps; allow foot back]

Left lower leg

Right upper leg [straighten knee, hard, and pull foot back toward the head; allow foot back]

Left upper leg

Scalp, forehead, and eyes [pull eyebrows down in a pretended angry frown while looking at an imaginary fly on your nose; feel a smooth wave of relaxation go over forehead and scalp while you look at the far horizon]

Cheeks [exaggerated "bad smell" look; allow cheeks to smooth out]

Mouth and tongue [ear to ear frog grin with tongue pressed against roof of the mouth; lips touching but loose and soft with teeth separated, tongue in middle of mouth]

Neck [pull head in like a turtle; allow head to be heavy]

Chest [push out chest; drop shoulders]

Abdomen [make stomach as rigid as a board; go soft]

Back [push yourself through the support behind you (floor or chair back); sit loose]

Buttocks and pelvic floor [bunch up as if stopping yourself from going to the bathroom; let it go]

For each muscle group, you go through a sequence that pairs the relaxation of the muscles with a key action and a key phrase. The best key action is to take a deep breath so that the stomach rises, and let it out slowly. The best key phrase (to think in your head) is "Let go" as you breathe out. Get into a quiet, comfortable position. Close your eyes and take a few deep breaths, then concentrate on the exercises. Breathe in, hold the tension, and *feel* it. Breathe out, say "Let go," and *feel* the difference.

Do each muscle group twice. Every now and then, go back and relax again a group you've dealt with. This means at least 32 pairings of relaxation with the signal.

The first session takes 15 to 20 minutes. Before getting up at the end, move around a little. Your blood pressure will have dropped, and if you stand up too suddenly you could feel dizzy and even fall.

Practice the sequence as often as possible, but at least once a day for two weeks. You will find that the sessions get shorter as you get better at it. You will be able to tense and relax bigger chunks of your body in one go (e.g., both arms together).

By the end of two weeks, you will be able to relax your whole body by letting go a single breath and thinking, "Let go!" Practice it in mild situations first. Each time the technique works, it gets stronger. If it ever fails, it gets weakened, and then you'll need to go back to more training sessions to restrengthen it.

Eventually, you can use it in difficult situations, like before an important exam or facing real physical danger or being furious and wanting to hit someone. It is unlikely to work once you are in the grip of strong emotion, but you can switch off the fear or anger *before* it takes full hold.

—Bob Rich, Ph.D.

■ ■ ■

I spent my nights reading all I could about the technology and the industry I had gotten myself into. It was a whole new language—point-to-point connectivity, line configurations, bandwidth, fiber optic networks. I had no practical knowledge of how any of these things worked, but I needed to understand enough to sound like I knew what I was talking about.

Though I was far from an overnight success, I did watch my successes grow. While others focused on gaining big accounts, I concentrated on doing as many sales calls as I could—50 a day was my goal. Smaller accounts were fine with me; even though they wouldn't earn me big commissions, they were easier to sell and meant that I had to talk to more people every day. Even though I hated doing it, that's just what I was there for. The more I could talk, the more I could build my self-esteem, and I could keep raising the bar for myself as I was able to handle more emotionally.

We had a philosophy at the company that people ultimately failed as sales reps for one of three reasons: lack of commitment, lack of capacity, or lack of skills and knowledge. The first two things had to come from within, and there wasn't much anyone could do to help you find them, but skills and knowledge could be improved just through steady effort and training. Anxiety disorders can work the same way.

I still saw the other reps and my bosses as the Michael Jordans of sales, though. They were the naturals, the aces. I was a scrappy kid who was playing dress-up and pretending I knew what "fiber optics" meant. Aside from weddings and funerals and fancy ceremonies, I had never worn a tie in my life.

About six months into the job, I found myself on the phone with the decision maker for McDonald's corporate office . . . now that would have been a large account! Actually, it would have been the biggest client our company had ever had—which is why everyone in the office hovered around me and listened as I spoke. I remember feeling apprehension and dread, like I was a guppy who somehow swam into killer whale territory . . . in the middle of a glass tank, so everyone could stare and point as I got mangled to bits. My sentences were quick, not well thought-out, nothing that would impress a powerhouse like McDonald's. They put me on hold a few times and I kept asking my boss for help. He told me, "This is sales, son . . . gotta be able to roll with the punches and think on your feet."

Having everyone judge my performance, scrutinizing me, was a worst-case scenario of mine. As I bombed, Ken was nice enough to take over, though he couldn't pick up the sale either. I looked great before the call, but horrible afterward because I caved under the pressure.

Sales taught me to fight continuously for rebounds, to come back stronger after defeat. I would not wallow in this lost opportunity for long. I often had five appointments a day and I couldn't allow one bad one to disrupt the rest. Anxiety was a roller coaster and I just had to accept that, ride it, and do the best I could in the present.

My coworkers often went out to lunch together, but I wasn't ready for that yet. I sat alone at my desk to eat, or I took my lunch on the road. They also socialized outside of work, and I never joined in. I couldn't, I rationalized, because all my free time was spent preparing for the next workday.

For at least an hour every night, I practiced my presentation. I videotaped myself and watched the playback to see where I could improve and what physical or vocal habits I needed to fix. I even practiced signing contracts—this always made me nervous in meetings, and I was convinced that you could make or break sales at this stage of the game.

Every month was a race to the quota line; I had to sell a certain number of phone lines, a certain number of accounts, a certain amount of revenue to live up to the company's goal and keep my job secure. I had the right determination, but one thing stood in the way of real progress in those early months. One desperate, wrong thought: "I *need* to make this sale!"

▪▪ 9 ▪▪

Self-Talk

Many persons have the wrong idea about what constitutes
true happiness. It is not attained through self-gratification
but through fidelity to a worthy purpose.
—HELEN KELLER

I had listened hard to mentors like Vince Lombardi, who often said,
"Winning isn't everything. It's the only thing." I listened so hard
that I still saw each meeting as a win/lose situation, all black-and-
white. If I didn't have the right sales numbers at the end of the
month, I was a failure.

My self-esteem was still conditional. *If* I gave a perfect presentation, and *if* I got that signed contract, then maybe I'd feel good about
myself that day, but by the next day I had already quit resting on my
laurels and felt I needed to prove myself again.

I saw myself as someone who had caught a lucky break—it just so
happened that the president of the company played basketball with
me, and it just so happened that my first sales manager was kind
enough to walk me through all those early meetings, and it just so
happened that my first role-play was cut off by that miraculous cell
phone call so I'd have a week to gather myself together and prepare.

God was looking out for me, sure, but what was going to happen if I didn't make those sales?

The bulk of my negative self-talk fell into the "What if?" category. What if I have a panic attack? What if I miss quota? What if I turn bright red in front of this businessman and he laughs at me? What if I forget my whole presentation and just wind up stammering and choking and drooling a little?

All of these "what ifs" turned into anticipatory anxiety. I'd anticipate feeling anxious or failing and I'd build up so much anxiety in my head that I was already panicking before I even started. And nearly every time, the horrors I imagined were far worse than what actually did happen. The things I worried about didn't come true— or if they did, they didn't warrant the kind of obsessive overthinking I had allocated to them. "What if I wind up foaming at the mouth and get carted away to an asylum?" never happened. But "What if I have a panic attack?" sometimes did. Even so, I'd spend two days freaking out with fear and making myself miserable over a problem that would last two minutes and probably not be noticed by anyone but myself.

"What if they think I'm stupid?" That thought kept me from asking others for help when I needed it. If I was confused at a meeting, I wouldn't speak up out of fear that people would look at me and think less of me for not understanding. Instead, I had to figure everything out on my own.

"What if I have a panic attack in front of a sales prospect? I have to do well or else I'm a loser. I'm weak." This kind of ultimatum didn't do me any good. It just added unreasonable pressure. I was always waiting for disaster to strike, always sure that it was just around the corner. It felt like I was swimming with sharks every day. One little blunder on my part would throw me into self-destruct mode.

Every day on the job, I would wake up filled with anxiety and put on my Joseph A. Banks pin-striped suit, a polo shirt (usually blue), and a dark-colored or silver tie. My new black wing-tip dress shoes pinched my toes as I walked miles and miles a day in them, going on cold calls. My feet were raw with blisters and my heels were cut up. All the way, I thought I was doing the right thing by not accepting failure and forcing myself to get out there. And all the way, I was thinking, "What if my voice cracks and I run out of air and I can't speak? I can't let that happen. I have to *sell*!"

Although what I was doing was probably an improvement over my attitude in my college days—I was now in the ring and fighting instead of just avoiding the world—it was still destructive. I was making my happiness conditional on almost random numbers and on outcomes that I couldn't control.

I couldn't control whether anyone ever bought anything from me. All I could do was prepare and work on my presentation; I couldn't force anyone to do anything, and even the best sales job in the world wouldn't convince some people to switch companies. So I had to quit focusing so hard on the results and instead focus on the effort.

I took Lombardi's "winning isn't everything" mantra, which was too perfectionistic for me, and modified it to suit my healthier attitude: "Effort isn't everything. It's the only thing."

Reprogramming my thoughts wasn't as easy as programming a new TV set, but just as methodical. I learned that, aside from the "what ifs," my negative thoughts fell into a few other categories: self-victimization, overgeneralization, catastrophic thinking, and underestimating myself.

When I felt particularly stung, I'd sometimes launch into victim mode, blaming everything in my life on this stupid anxiety disorder. "Why me? It's not fair!" The truth is that anxiety sure isn't any fun, but it can be there to teach us important lessons and help us improve our lives rather than destroy us. I couldn't go back and change the past, so I couldn't stop the anxiety disorder from coming on. There was no use in getting stuck in self-pity for very long. I didn't choose to get an anxiety disorder, but I did have the power to choose how to deal with it and how to respond to it . . . as well as what lessons I would take away from it.

If I had a bad experience in one situation, I would assume it was going to happen that way every time. I didn't feel good about the way I had interacted with women since the panic had started, so I just avoided dating, thinking I would always do poorly with women. "I'll say something stupid," I thought. And if I had a panic attack in a certain restaurant or store, I didn't want to return there, because my brain told me that I was always going to have trouble in those places.

Catastrophizing seemed to come easy for me. "I am messed up and will be like this forever." When that popped up in my journal—which was often, in various forms—I had to remember to counter it with more rational thoughts: "My condition is temporary. If I prepare as well as I possibly can and commit to work on this plan for recovery, I will be fine. Millions of people have suffered from this and gotten better. I am not a freak. It's common to feel this way and everybody has to go through adversity. I welcome this as an opportunity to grow and become stronger. I will not die from this. My symptoms will be uncomfortable, but as I grow day by day, my fears and symptoms will gradually subside as well."

■ ■ ■

In their book *Painfully Shy*, the Markways recommend examining the validity of your negative thoughts. Test them against the following questions:

- What is the evidence that this statement is true?
- Who says it's true?
- What gives him or her the right to decide it's true?
- So what if it's true? Does it matter?

■ ■ ■

Social anxiety and panic made me learn to doubt myself. I had lost belief in my talents and abilities, and it would take a lot of retraining to bring me back to a point where I could maintain eye contact and feel equal to others. Very rarely did I compare myself favorably to other people, and I was always trying to measure up to people I thought were innately better than I was—more confident, more polished, smarter, savvier. When I walked into those early sales calls, I felt inferior to everyone I approached. I had trouble speaking up and am surprised I made sales at all. But I learned to give myself pep talks to counter my negative thoughts before going into a sales meeting.

"This guy may be a tough business guy, but I can slam dunk in his face. He is no better than I am. I am calm and confident and I am prepared for this meeting." I tried to look self-assured long before I truly was. Psychologists say that you should act as if you are already where you want to be, and the reality will follow your act.

I put my negative thoughts and worries against a "So what?" test. If my worry was that I was going to have a red face, I'd ask myself, "So? I'll have a red face. Big deal. Doesn't make me a bad person. Besides, in my whole life, only one or two people have ever commented that my face was red. People probably won't even notice, and if they do, they won't think I'm nuts just because of that." If the thought was, "What if I panic?" I could counter it with, "So? Nobody is perfect; everyone goes through their own challenges."

■ ■ ■

I recommend that when people are starting to work with self-talk they spend half an hour each day writing and countering fearful self-statements for about two weeks. After you've done this a dozen times or so, the process starts to internalize. The shortcut approach is to put positive self-talk or affirmations on an audiotape and listen to the tape each day for a couple of weeks. It's normal to feel that the whole process of writing everything down is "cheesy" or contrived in the beginning.

—Edmund J. Bourne, Ph.D.

■ ■ ■

It was hard not to get caught up in my day-to-day worries, but I was trying to focus on the big picture: my long-term goal of living a life without limits. That meant that I had to practice the fundamentals every day until they became instinctual.

No matter how miserable I felt, on the way in to work, I would run through affirmations and positive self-talk. "I can't wait to face the day! I am going to grow today, no matter what happens. It's all good. I am going to give the best presentation ever today!" Many of the comments felt "cheesy," but they helped me brainwash myself by pushing back all of the detrimental thoughts.

I even had to learn how to reinterpret my own body signals. To me, heart racing meant an impending heart attack, and a shot of adrenaline in my gut meant I was afraid and couldn't handle the situation. I had to learn to quit seeing each symptom as scary and unbeatable. I couldn't make the feelings stop, so I had to do something about how I responded to them.

It may sound crazy, but I decided to induce panic attacks on purpose, just so I could prove to myself that nothing terrible would ever result from them. Before a sales meeting, I would run up and down stairs to get my heart racing, which was one of my panic warning signs. Then I'd just rush into the office out of breath.

It's like a basketball team preparing for a full court press. In basketball, there are five players per side. We often prepared for a full court press by playing against seven or eight swarming defenders as a way of creating focus so we would be ready for the frenzy. It's the same with panic. I had to get used to the chaos and find a way to use it to my advantage.

Sometimes the thoughts would creep up: "I'm having a heart attack! I'm going to faint! I'm going to die!"

None of those things ever happened and I kept reminding myself of this until I believed it. No matter how bad my symptoms felt, I would always get through them, and there wouldn't be any permanent damage or risk to my health. Maybe I could even use them to my benefit the way great actors actually gain from stage fright: the adrenaline makes their performances even more exciting and energetic. They are truly in the moment and performing their hearts out. If they failed to get nervous anymore, their performances would probably be lackluster and routine. My sales job was similar; I learned to interpret the heart-racing and sweaty palms as signs that I was ready and about to put on a good show.

My biggest fear before a meeting was that I would have a panic attack and run out of air. By running up stairs, I was already out of air before the meeting began. I prepared myself for the feeling and went through with it. "Take that, fear. What else have you got?"

Slowly, I gained more confidence as I went on these sales calls, and I made my quota every month. Maybe I wasn't the misfit in a company of outstanding sales reps, after all. Maybe we were all human and maybe other people felt scared too and had their own obstacles to overcome.

Initially, when I wrote down positive thoughts to counter my negative thoughts, I didn't always trust them. When I thought, "I am crazy" and countered it with, "I am a perfectly sane person who is just going through a hard time right now, but I'm working on it and I'm improving every day," I didn't wholeheartedly believe myself. I made a point of not coming up with over-the-top, completely unbelievable replacement thoughts, but I still had some convincing to do.

■ ■ ■

I suggest that we need not only to tune into our negative self-talk but to go one step further and apologize to ourselves. After all, we would never speak as cruelly to other people as we do to ourselves. If we did say something hurtful to a friend, we'd certainly apologize. So we should do the same for ourselves.

I know this might seem awkward at first, but we need to give ourselves the same respect that we give others. For example, you might say something (this could be silently, aloud, or written in a journal) like, "I'm sorry I keep saying mean things. Just because you get nervous doesn't mean you're a loser. You're kind and sensitive and have a lot to offer. You deserve to be happy and feel loved."

—Barbara G. Markway, Ph.D.

■ ■ ■

For example, I wouldn't replace the "I am crazy" thought with "I'm perfect and I'm the smartest, most sane, most worthy person in the world." Some people think you need to puff yourself up with grandiose thoughts that are the polar opposite of your negative thoughts, but that's not true. It does you no good to ignore the nuggets of truth in your negative thoughts: No, I wasn't crazy, but I also didn't need to pretend that my life was perfect and that I had nothing to improve upon. There was a reason for that negative thought in the first place, so I had to address it in my new response.

"Yes, I was having problems, but I am taking the right steps and working hard to defeat my problems." That was a positive thought without being too outrageous to swallow. Even so, in the early stages, I didn't always accept these positive thoughts right away. "Yeah, sure," I'd think. "I don't feel like I'm getting better every day. In fact, today I feel like crawling into a hole and never coming out. So who cares how hard I'm working?"

One of the keys to reprogramming the way your brain works is repetition and consistency. You must keep challenging those thoughts, not once in a while or when you happen to notice, but every time, possibly for weeks, months, or years until you don't have to keep doing it because those negative thoughts don't even bother to show up anymore. Once they know they've been defeated, they won't stick around to keep getting beat down. They'll just slink off quietly and let the positive thoughts claim their victory.

■ ▒ ■

He was really flooding his mind with positive talk. He had all these quotes he'd written down. He'd be reading this when he went to sleep at night; he'd read it in the morning. He made copies for me so I knew them. He practiced his pitch with his mom, to the mirror at night . . .

To me, it looked a lot like how an athlete would prepare for an intense event. Every day, every meeting he walked into was like how I would look at a game. All of the positive quotes and stuff—that's what coaches fill your head with. And Jamie was constantly reviewing his game plan. That way, when he went into a meeting he knew it cold and didn't have to think to go through it. It was second nature.

—Brian Musso (old friend)

■ ■ ■

And so it was that I not only survived in the high-pressure sales world, but I thrived. I think that my insecurities worked in my favor because they made me human and a good listener; I didn't come off as a slick salesman. My talent, which took me months to realize, is that I was able to connect with people—to ask questions that showed I cared about their businesses, to make small talk, to disarm people with humor. Once, when a man asked me what problems he could expect when he switched from another company to ours, I responded, "Well, the fire alarms will go off and your entire building will be flooded with water. We have a monkey that will reside in the telecom room in case of emergency." Never underestimate the power of making people laugh.

I also gave myself an "out." I gave myself permission to leave if things ever got too overwhelming. It was okay to go to the bathroom to take a break or to walk out of the building for air or even to go home early if need be. And if things ever fell apart, I told myself I could just bolt to L.A., where no one would know me. This was pure fantasy and of course I never did it, but it worked. A lot of pressure lifted when I told myself I would not be a failure and I would not be angry with myself if I had to leave. Just knowing I always had an escape available made me much more comfortable and able to take bigger risks.

When I felt like I was going to lose it on sales calls, I knew I had to interrupt my fearful thoughts. I've heard of some people who keep a rubber band around their wrists and snap it when a fearful thought intrudes. I wasn't quite as literal about "snapping out of it," but I would pinch my leg as hard as I could under the table. This would focus me on the present and take my mind off its worrying.

In a business where 95 percent of our efforts are met with rejection, many get demoralized. I learned how to handle rejection by staring it in the face every day, by looking at a big whiteboard that showed the names of each rep and how they were doing that month for all in the office to see and judge, and by pounding the pavement and having doors slammed in my face. Rather than dwelling on the rejections, I saw each doorway as a new opportunity to get better at my presentation and become more prepared, both for this career and for the world at large.

I had my share of setbacks and embarrassments—like when I was so nervous at a meeting that I bit my pen until it exploded in my mouth, which I didn't realize until the client pointed out that my mouth was blue, or when I leaned back in my chair so far that it flipped over during a presentation—but I actually made my quotas and I felt I was on the right track.

Then one morning, five and a half months after I began my sales job and just as I was finding a level of comfort and satisfaction from it, I walked into work and found out that my mentor, Ken, was gone. He was moved to another role in the organization and he was to be replaced by a man named Sam Snair.

I got chills when I typed that last sentence. I have never feared anyone in my life as much as I feared Sam Snair. He arrived like a human jackhammer, about to take every inch of my newly formed foundation and try to bust it up into fragments and dust. The test of my survival was about to start. And I was one minute late for it.

▪▪ IO ▪▪

The Trial

Obstacles cannot crush me. Every obstacle yields to stern
resolve. He who is fixed to a star does not change his mind.
—Leonardo da Vinci

On the wall behind his desk was a picture of a grizzly bear sinking
its long, bloody fangs into a defenseless salmon. It was probably the
first thing he moved into his office, and very quickly, I understood
why he identified with the picture. In fact, every time I saw his face,
the outline of that image burned into my retina. He was the bear; we
were the salmon.

I walked in at 7:01 that morning and Snair just stared at me as I
made my way to my cube. He sauntered over and just stared at me in
silence. After a minute or so, he said, "You're late," in a slow, deep,
Clint Eastwood voice. "It's 7:01 and you have to be here at 7:00. If it
happens again, you're fired." Then he leaned in closely to whisper
choice expletives and threats: "Man, I'll put you on that wall; I'll
have you looking down that wall; I'll knock you off that bleeping
wall," he said.

He walked back to his office, reveling in the fear he'd just stirred
up, and I sat dumbfounded. I wasn't the only one. At the end of
Snair's first month, 10 sales reps had quit under the intense pressure.

He didn't have to fire anyone; he just created enough chaos, disharmony, and cruelty that people wilted under him and left on their own.

Snair's presence dominated before he even spoke. His greatest talent was keeping people off balance, never knowing what was coming next from him. On rare days, he'd act like your best friend. The rest of the time, he sought to break people down, intimidate us, and humiliate us. I once overheard him say that if you beat people down like dogs, they'll bend to your will. He wanted to build up a sales force that would fear and worship him.

Ken had been about empowerment and professionalism; Snair believed in humiliation and dictatorship. He'd even tell us, "No matter what you've heard, all men are not all created equal. Some of us are better than others. This is not a damn democracy. I make the rules."

Each morning, he'd bring us into his office and we'd go around the room, one at a time, explaining what we had accomplished the day before. You could smell the fear in that room.

We sat there with frozen faces, sullen, numb, as if he were Medusa turning us to stone. If you didn't live up to his expectations each day—oh, and by the way, he had immediately doubled our quotas to make them the highest in the industry—you could expect to face his unabashed wrath and ridicule. You didn't want to be the one who fell short.

Those morning meetings were more agonizing than going for root canal every single day. I always felt on the verge of collapse around Snair, and what's worse is that I knew how much he was enjoying it. He called me a slacker, a gutless turd. He said I was weak and not cut out for this job. Told me he had bets on when I was going to quit—he wagered that I'd last only a few more days.

The way things were going, I thought he might just win that bet. He would put job applications to fast food restaurants on my desk and tell me I'd be in a mental hospital or doing his landscaping before he was through with me. He broke into my e-mail and told people I was moving to San Francisco to marry my gay lover.

On more than one occasion, he said I had been coat-tailing my old manager Ken—asking Ken to step in whenever anything got tough. Of course, he may have been right—but he had no idea why I needed that help, and I wasn't about to open my heart to him. I think he saw me as a "teacher's pet," and he was determined to show me that things would be different now . . . much different.

Snair had imported his friends into the company. He had a few favorites whom he'd conditioned over the years, and while they lacked his strength, they shared his craftiness. All the leads went to them. Their salaries were higher and their promotions came easily, even when I outperformed them.

He lived inside my head, working hard to reverse all the positive self-talk I had practiced. He told me I didn't have what it took. I was worthless. I had been coddled, but now I could no longer suck on my mom's breast. (He actually said that in more vulgar terms.) And as much as I wanted to kill him for all his insults and nasty treatment, I barely said a word. I just thought that if I could meet his inhuman expectations, maybe he'd grow to respect me.

Meanwhile, I was in for the greatest trial I had faced since the panic began. I had been getting better and better, building momentum and gaining confidence, and then this guy showed up. It would have been much easier to leave and find myself a new job, but somewhere within, I knew I had to rise to this challenge and come out on top. I could not let this man win. I could not let him break me.

My daily goal increased. Instead of going on 50 cold calls a day, now I went on 75, which lasted morning through evening. Snair checked my activity reports daily, calling a few of my prospects every day to make sure I had really been there. And I made sales. I hit my quota every month, but rarely received any praise for it. It's lucky that I wasn't dependent on praise to keep me going. Not that I would have minded a few nice comments, of course, but his no-excuses attitude forced me to challenge my fears even more—which I knew I needed to do, even if I hated every minute of it.

If you missed your quota two or three months in a row, you got fired. Even if you hit 99 percent of your quota each month. You could be the biggest stud in the world, but you still had to start at zero every month. From the first day of the month to the last, I never let my head get big or my status get too cushy. There were a few months when I was down to the last day, the last hour, and I was still just shy of my quota. Miracles came through in the eleventh hour time and again because I didn't give up or crack. I just kept making phone calls until something came through.

I heard grown men talking to themselves at their desks, sweating and crying from the pressure. It was strange to me that these people—those whom I saw as icons and models of professional businesspeople—cracked sooner than I did.

That's not to say I rose above it all without difficulty. No, I had many sleepless nights where I'd just sit in bed and stare at the walls, feeling like the air had been sucked out of the room, and dreading the tyrannical eye of daybreak. I sometimes did fall apart with panic in sales meetings.

Every meeting, I was on the brink of an attack. It was a waiting game to see how bad it would get. If the attacks were moderate, I'd do my best to sit and suffer through them. If they went over the top to desperation, I'd make an excuse to leave, telling the potential client that I was late to a meeting and would come back later. I know I lost sales because of it.

My bosses often listened in on my phone calls, and it nearly drove me mad. And coworkers would eavesdrop openly. Our cubicles had the feel of an egg carton: We were all right next to one another, breathing down each other's neck. I used to take my stuff and go to an empty office to make my calls, telling them I could focus better that way. The truth was that I feared their judgment.

So I continued working on my speaking skills, reading the paper aloud just to hear how I sounded to myself. I would turn on the closed captioning on my TV and read it like a teleprompter. Even when I least wanted to, I made small talk with strangers in stores, trying to learn how to build rapport. When you have social anxiety disorder, it can be hard to talk about yourself, so I focused on the other person, asking lots of questions. Most people love talking about themselves anyway.

Snair became the embodiment of all of my fears. All of those niggling doubts I had about myself, he expressed and exploited, usually in front of everybody. The one thing I had going for me was my growing career success, and it seemed that he tried to undermine that at every turn. He belittled my work, but I didn't quit. I won trips to Florida, Hawaii, and the Bahamas for being a top salesman. At the end of 1998, my first full year on the job, I was the company's top Chicago rep: Salesman of the Year.

The night I received that award, I lay in my bed doing Tiger Woods–like fist pumps, saying, "I did it! I can't believe I did it!"

My fear had driven me to great lengths, and I was growing into a top-notch sales rep, outperforming people who were twice my age and had far more experience in telecom. My goals shifted, and I was no longer satisfied with just getting by; now I had visions of excellence. When I walked out of an office, I wanted the boss to say, "That was the best salesman I've ever seen."

I hit my quota 18 months in a row, a company record. The person who had come the closest had only met quota for six or seven months consecutively. But the problem was that I let this quota consume me. Somewhere, I lost track of my "big picture" and I became a little too fond of the money and the bragging rights.

When complaints came in, I ignored them. Clients would sometimes have problems with their phone lines, and because I sold them the products, I was to blame. I often avoided those calls, procrastinating in the hopes that if I ignored them, they'd go away. Yeah, that wasn't such a great strategy. And I learned that the more I procrasti-nated, the more my anxiety built. Much better to face the music and get it over with. Dealing with adversity head-on was a skill I still had to master.

And adversity was in no short supply. I was staring adversity in the face every day, in the form of my arch nemesis Snair. He'd give me an order and I'd tell him I'd get it done. "Now . . . right *now*," he'd command, then proceed to insult my work ethic in words I can't repeat in polite company.

But in the second week of February 1999, he shocked me. I had begun the new year with a bang—220 percent over quota in the first month, and I'd be at 80 percent of my quota today with plenty of time to spare. All I had to do was pick up a contract from a client who'd called to tell me it was signed. I had already gone out for some drinks with friends the night before to celebrate. Maybe a few too many drinks. As I was about to leave my horribly cramped cubicle, Snair walked over and asked, "Wanna grab some lunch?"

This man had performed relentless and ruthless psychological torture on me for eight months, and now he wanted to go out to lunch? I was stunned. His voice had even transformed from formi-dable to almost friendly. "My treat," he said. "You've been working your ass off, and you said you were picking up a big deal today. In my book, that's grounds for some grub."

I couldn't have been more shocked if the Swedish bikini team showed up and offered to tune my car. Was he really being nice, or was this some twisted plan to ultimately break me down? As much as I would have liked to call a cease-fire with him, I couldn't take the risk of sitting one-on-one with him. His presence was ominous to me, and if anybody could induce a panic attack, it was he. Every time he came near me, I had to fight back tears and work on keeping my heart steady.

"Thanks, Sam, but I have to go pick up that deal," I said.

"Cool, man. Go knock it down and take the rest of the day off. You may even be able to catch some soaps or Springer if you're lucky."

I laughed nervously and thanked him. And just when I thought I was off the hook . . . "Hey, your meeting is at 35 East Wacker. I have a client I have to see there. Let's catch a cab, you pick up your deal, and we'll meet in the lobby afterwards. I'll process the paperwork for you and you can take off."

This level of kindness was wholly new to me. Maybe my sentence of punishment was over. The cab ride would be only a few minutes, and I figured that I could handle that.

We made it to the building and parted ways. I was to see Mr. Jameson, the CEO of an insurance company. We had already met three times and now all I had to do was pick up that signed contract. Easy stuff—no selling, no negotiating. I felt good until I got crammed into an elevator filled with business executives for 52 floors. My heart sped up and tension shot through my stomach, mounting with each floor.

Because of my panic attacks, I overreacted to the slightest shift in my physiology and couldn't take my focus off it. I tried to calm myself with encouraging thoughts: "I can do this. Get a grip! I am relaxed, I am relaxed." I took deep, slow breaths from my abdomen, but it seemed that the more I tried, the worse I got. Sweat trickled down my blue dress shirt, my hands got cold and clammy, and my muscles felt tight. The "what ifs" won the day this time.

"What if I have a panic attack and lose it in the meeting? He'll think I'm nuts and there won't be any escape. I'll lose the sale. And how will I face Snair? He'll humiliate me at our next meeting and I'll finally have a complete breakdown. He'll humiliate me in front of everybody! I'll miss quota this month. One more month and he'll fire me!" The thoughts raced by quicker than I could counter them, and my face burned as if on fire.

■ ■ ■

It is usually hard for people with anxiety disorders to learn to relax because they have mistakenly learned to associate hypervigilant, hyperaroused, and hyperdefensive psychophysiological (mind-body) states with being in control. This becomes the problem! It is imperative to break this reflex with learning to "let go," which is an integration of emotional trust and physical relaxation. The most effective relaxation technique I have used is based on biofeedback training. The objective and scientific measurement provided by the machines greatly facilitates the awareness/learning process. A very powerful strategy is the learning of hand warming, which is conscious vasodilation of the blood vessels leading to increased peripheral blood flow. The ability to raise the skin temperature of one's hand three to four degrees can abort an anxiety attack.

—Jonathan Berent, A.C.S.W.

■ ■ ■

Mr. Jameson greeted me with a handshake and warm smile. "Great to see you again, Jamie! Let's wrap this up." I was overly aware that my handshake must have felt like holding a clammy fish.

We had built up a great affinity over the past three meetings and had common interests from basketball to movies. He trusted me, and I liked him.

"Did you catch the Bulls game the other night against the Miami Heat? Jordan went for that circus shot and Alonzo took his feet out from under him . . . I hope we meet those guys in the playoffs. Matter of fact, I have tickets to the game next week against Shaq. My daughter is going with me. Want to tag along? She's a beautiful girl, played basketball in college. Bet she could give you a run for your money."

His daughter's picture was behind him on the wall and he was grinning widely, expecting my enthusiasm. She was a young, golden-haired stunner with a self-assured smile, and I suddenly felt like Gollum from *Lord of the Rings*. The easy meeting was turning out to be anything but; my mind swarmed with a thousand flashing thoughts—none of them any good. "This nice guy is trying to be friendly and even set me up with his gorgeous, smart daughter, and I'm freaking out! He's going to find out what a loony tune I am, and then he'll back out of the deal. Sooner or later I'll crack . . . hell, I'm cracking up now!"

I squirmed in my chair, clutching the handrails as if I were trying to break them, bracing myself for the impending onslaught. My heart leapt in my chest . . . fast, fast, fast. The room went blurry and I couldn't compose myself.

My eyes watered and it took all the strength I had to hold myself together. "Uh, I have to eat at my relatives' that night, but thanks for offering," I stammered, trying to catch my breath.

"Maybe some other time," he said.

My eyes darted around the room like a frightened animal, and I scanned my brain for an appropriate response, but words escaped me. Everything felt distorted and tense. I was certain he could see that I was falling apart.

"All right, let's get down to business," he said.

He handed me the contract, and it was, indeed, signed. Thank God, I thought. Just hold on two more minutes and you're out of here. Home free.

"I just have one question about the contract. It says it automatically renews in a year. What if I don't want to renew?"

Having been asked that question a hundred times already, I knew exactly the right answer, but it refused to come out of my mouth. My voice shook and cracked and I responded as briefly as possible, about one step away from caveman grunts.

"Do you want some water?" he asked.

"Yes, yes, get me some f#@*&^ water! Give me a reprieve from this hell," I wanted to reply, but managed to choke out, "Sure."

He came back with a cup of water, then jumped back in with questions. "How do you explain how the network is designed to interface with the incumbent network?"

He was testing me. He had already asked me the same question a few weeks back, but this time, when I answered, sweat ran down my face and my words were jumbled. It looked like I was lying. Trust is paramount in sales, and I knew I was creating doubt in this man's mind with my shifty reactions.

My resolve expired. When he asked further questions, even when I knew the answers, I just said, "I don't know." This was the white flag of surrender. If I uttered another sentence, I was going to cry. Normally, I would have fought for that sale, but not today. Today, panic was the stronger opponent.

Mr. Jameson saved me by saying, "Tell you what, Jamie . . . can you give me another week to look this over? Thanks, buddy."

I shook his hand and walked out of the office with my head down, anxiety fading into a shallow hopelessness. I had blown it—that sale wasn't coming back.

But the worst of it wasn't over. The worst of it was waiting for me in the lobby with the expectation of a signed contract for 60 phone lines. On the elevator, I sank deeper into myself with each descending floor, anticipating the wrath that awaited me.

"Let's see the goods," Snair said.

"I lost the deal," I said quietly. "Well, I didn't definitely lose it, but he wants more time."

"Good, I'm proud of you," he shot back with sarcasm. Then he stood and stared at me in silence, forcing me to feel the awkward tension he thrived on. We weren't even out the door before he let loose with a torrent of invectives.

"You said it was a done deal! Kind of arrogant, don't you think? You have two weeks to make up your quota. You'll be out of here before you know it, and you know what? It's for your own good. You can't hack it. Nobody thinks you're going to make it; they all think you've been lucky. I believed in you, but my patience with you is up. Time is ticking."

He fumed the whole way back in the cab, cursing out the driver and random pedestrians on the street for good measure.

Once away from his brutal presence, I went for a walk and bought some coffee. I usually bought decaf, but at this point, did it really matter?

∎ ∎ ∎

People with anxiety disorders should avoid any foods or drinks that tend to cause the same feelings associated with panic attacks. Caffeine may cause jitteriness and anxiousness. Alcohol can cause lightheaded feelings. Also, skipping meals can cause lightheadedness and low blood sugar, which could cause someone to break out in sweats and feel like they're going to pass out.

—Heidi (Reichenberger) McIndoo, M.S., R.D., L.D.N.

∎ ∎ ∎

The Chicago air hovered around zero, and I filled my deprived lungs with its chill. Fresh white snow covered the earth like a quilt. I couldn't help but notice how the world seemed so still, so peaceful— so much the opposite of everything I was feeling inside. Shameful, pathetic. The game was on the line and I choked. Chaos created a persistent buzz in my head, telling me I was ugly and useless. I wanted to leave, to be anywhere but here.

"All this hard work I've done, it's all amounted to nothing!" I thought. "I was supposed to be better now! I was supposed to be rid of these stupid attacks. I'm never going to be normal. My life is always going to be a prison."

On my way in to work at 6:30 the next morning, I found myself making a U-turn, unwilling to show up for my crucifixion at Snair's meeting. I called in sick, and Snair told me I had to come in if I wanted to keep my job. I said I would try, but that I was throwing up and probably couldn't. He didn't believe me, of course—"It's okay if you want to quit," he said, but I told him weakly that I wanted to stay.

■ ■ ■

Putting yourself in situations wherein you experience your fear and cope with it is essential to your recovery. You should do it in a controlled, systematic fashion as often as possible. However, it is not necessary to do this 24/7. We all need a break now and then to recharge our batteries. Whether you are socially anxious, shy, introverted, or hypersensitive to stimuli, you will tend to find social interaction wearing rather than energizing. As a result, you will need to have time away from social interaction to collect your thoughts and regroup.

However, at the same time, it is important that this natural need for a 'time out' is not overdone and used as an excuse for avoidance of feared situations. By making daily entries in your journal about anxiety instances, when and where they occur, and how you react to them, you can look for behavior patterns and monitor whether you are escaping rather than recuperating.

—Signe Dayhoff, Ph.D.

■ ■ ■

The words were only half-true. Maybe I should just quit, I told myself. I didn't leave my bed all day and night. On Saturday, I finally moved to the couch and flipped to a program about Martin Luther King. King was on a peaceful march to advocate nonviolent resistance in the town of Cicero, Illinois, 15 minutes from where I lived. Back then, Cicero was a town brimming with racism and hate, and King said in an interview that he thought this would be his last day on earth. Nevertheless, he marched. He marched beside banners that read, "Kill King! Wipe them out! Exterminate blacks!" He marched when a firework went off and he grabbed his side, thinking he had been shot. He marched when someone threw a brick that hit him in the head. The blow knocked him to the ground, but he arose slowly, covered in blood. A doctor told him to go to the hospital for stitches, but King said he wanted to keep marching, even if it meant his own death.

Keep marching.

After the program, I picked up a book I had been meaning to read: *Man's Search for Meaning* by Viktor Frankl, a Jewish psychologist who survived a Nazi concentration camp. He described in horrific detail the sleeping quarters where prisoners alive and dead were stacked on top of each other. They were given numbers instead of names, worked in the snow for the Nazi regime while battling frostbite and starvation, forced to watch their loved ones die in gas chambers. Husbands were ordered to kill their wives and children. The stench of gas and smoke and death hovered everywhere.

Frankl's whole family was killed, but he somehow survived by finding meaning despite the horrors he was forced to live with. When people tried to steal his food, he'd give it away. "Everything can be taken from a man but . . . the last of human freedoms . . . to choose one's attitude in any given set of circumstances, to choose one's way." He watched men who had given up hope fall gravely ill or kill themselves. One of his fellow prisoners had a dream where a voice told him he'd be free on March 30. The man was very excited and happy, but as the time grew closer and nothing changed, he lost hope. On March 29, he became very ill. On the 30th, he became delirious and passed out, and he died the following day. The story reminded me how powerful a positive vision is. Without it, we die . . . if not physically, then at least spiritually.

Although Frankl wasn't in good health, he had to fake it and appear as if he was or else he was dead. But he saw each day of survival as a victory, and turned his misery into optimism.

On that Saturday, Martin Luther King and Viktor Frankl saved my life. If these men could find strength in the worst possible conditions, then I could too. They put my troubles into perspective for me and convinced me to fight another day. I would never be able to control the demands of my work or my boss, but I could choose my response to the fear they created. Life was going to go on.

Five Minutes Longer

A hero is no braver than an ordinary man,
but he is braver five minutes longer.
—RALPH WALDO EMERSON

There were a mop and bucket next to my desk, and my nametag had been replaced by the custodian's. Applications to landscaping companies and burger joints sat on my chair, and my computer screen was filled with question marks, as if to say, "Is he going to make it?" Snair had sent one of his lackeys to do this while he was ripping my head off my neck in his office. He thought this was it, that he finally had me licked. I erased the question marks from the screen, gathered my essentials into my briefcase, and walked out the door.

What might have been fear and humiliation turned into fury and a laser-beam focus. I peeled out in my car and headed to a large business building in the city, where I was determined to cover the first 10 floors—even if I didn't leave until midnight.

I barged into the first door and found an office with 30 people behind desks. Nobody looked up. Loudly, so everyone could hear, I announced, "Sorry to bother you all, but I need to talk with whoever handles your telecommunications decisions." The humming of activity stopped and all eyes were on me. Normally, I would have caved, but today, I wasn't giving my anxiety even an inch of space.

The workers looked at me as if I were the most abject person they had ever laid eyes on, and I repeated myself. I was usually more polite, asking if it would be possible to talk to the person, or "I'd really appreciate it if I could talk . . ." But today I was the revolting sales guy everyone hates, and I was not backing down.

A man stood up at the back of the room. "How can I help you? What are you selling?" he asked with an expression that told me no matter what I said, he wasn't buying. I told him who I was and what I was offering, and instead of asking for an appointment to speak with him at his convenience, I stood there and started my spiel right on the spot. I needed sales, and I needed them now.

We must have looked like a theatrical performance, with both of us standing in the middle of the room challenging each other and matching wits. For once, I just didn't care that 30 people were watching me potentially make a fool of myself.

He finally agreed to listen, and I took a maverick approach. Right at his desk, I called the customer service numbers of other companies and got put on hold by a machine. I called our customer service number and got through to a human being in 10 seconds. I called customers and asked them to provide references to this guy on the spot. Then I wrote up a proposal that showed how we could save him thousands of dollars. Not only did he sign, but he also signed another contract for the business's second location in the suburbs.

The next morning at our meeting, Snair looked astounded when I walked in—he was sure he'd seen the last of me. But he feigned indifference and went on with business. He'd set up a contest: whoever had sold the most revenue the day before would get tickets to the Bulls game that night. He knew that one of his buddies had sold a good amount, and just as he was about to hand him the tickets, I asked, "How much is your account?"

The guy said, "Let's see your deal first."

I threw my contract on the table. To Snair's delight, the guy exclaimed, "I gotcha by two grand, chump!"

Then I threw my second contract down. Oh, sweet victory.

When Snair begrudgingly handed me my tickets, he warned me not to stay out and drink because it wouldn't be in my best interest to be late the next day.

I called my brother to invite him to the game. In my new red Acura, I cranked up some Springsteen and slipped briefly out of the world of sales and Snair and panic. Today, I won. The Sears Tower loomed over the city, planted against a backdrop of steel darkness and bright white stars. The city danced with light that night. It hit me that this was the game Mr. Jameson had invited me to attend with his daughter. Maybe I would see them there after all.

Over the next year, I learned to trust in my abilities. One bad day could not negate all of the progress I had made, and I began standing up for myself with increasing regularity. Although Snair remained my adversary, I learned to use his harsh rants to my benefit. I grew strong, battle-ready, self-reliant, and thick-skinned. Just as he accepted no excuses from me, I accepted no excuses from myself.

When I looked back on that lost sale, I was able to recognize why it happened. As important as it is to celebrate successes, it's also important to examine failures and figure out what went wrong. Why did I fail? What could I have done differently? Was I prepared? What were my emotions and thoughts like? What actions can I take right now to improve? Though I had never become complacent—panic wouldn't allow that—I had eased up on my Panic Plan after a good run of success. I found answers to my questions: I had gone out drinking the night before and awakened late that day. I hadn't prepared myself for questions as I usually did, and Snair's presence in the building set me on edge. When I went in to pick up the contract, my motivation was money, not growth.

Adversity can set the stage for improvement if you can shift your focus from the problem to the solution. Okay, so I had a setback, but now I had the option to choose how to react to it. It reminded me of an interview with Tiger Woods after he hit an amazing shot through narrow trees and onto the green. The reporter asked how he made it through the trees. Tiger answered, "What trees? I was focusing on the opening."

It was time to get back to the fundamentals again, to the things that led to my success in the first place. I inspired myself again with positive self-talk and affirmations. I exercised and stayed away from food and drinks with high sugar and caffeine. I practiced my presentation and researched the answers to questions I was still unsure about. Proving people wrong when they've underestimated me is a big joy of mine. In this case, Snair lit a fire in me and I had to bring out my best.

▪ ▪ ▪

In addition to avoiding caffeine and alcohol, it's important for those with anxiety to eat regularly throughout the day. Don't go longer than three to four hours without eating. And, as much as possible, have each meal or snack be a combination of lean protein, such as fish, chicken, low-fat milk, yogurt or cheese, eggs, nuts and nut butters, and complex carbohydrates, such as whole grain breads, crackers, cereals, and fruits. These carbs provide energy, and the protein prolongs feelings of fullness and helps keep blood sugar levels on an even keel.

—Heidi (Reichenberger) McIndoo, M.S., R.D., L.D.N.

▪ ▪ ▪

I had fallen backward a bit with my anxiety disorder, but now I would quit focusing on the outcome and instead go back to focusing on the things I could control: my attitude and preparation.

Some people think that you're either born an optimist or a pessimist, and that's that. But I defied that. My father was a cynical guy and so was I. You really can change your outlook on life just by consciously working on it, by choosing a new attitude and practicing that attitude until you master it.

Snair challenged me to push myself to my outer limits. He made my life miserable sometimes, but without him, I'm not sure if I would have progressed as well as I did. I had to earn every small measure of success, and if I screwed up, no one was going to pat my head and tell me it was okay.

And I knew that when, a few months later in June, I missed my quota for the first time in 18 months. Not only did I fail, but I failed spectacularly, only hitting about 5 percent of the target. I did it on purpose.

That month I purposely didn't make any new sales. I researched and worked on accounts I had already landed, but I decided not to turn in any new deals . . . yet. When Snair asked me what was going on, I kept telling him I had all kinds of accounts in the pipeline.

No matter how much he acted like he hated me (and he probably did), I still made Snair's job easier. He knew he could count on my making that quota month after month. He had repeatedly told me that he'd promote me to senior account executive when I was ready for it, which meant a higher salary—and a higher quota, making it easier to fail. I knew what was behind his scheme. He would put more pressure on me and have more control and I would break.

But on this particular June morning, I quit caring. I had turned the corner and vowed not to let Snair run my life. I had come too far for that. So that day, I decided not to come through on his terms. I came through on my own terms instead.

It was June 30, the last day of the month—which meant the last day for me to make up that missing 95 percent of my quota. I struck a friendship with the owner of a large corporation and sold an account. But I asked the guy to tell a white lie for me: "If my boss calls," I said, "would you tell him you signed the deal on July 1 and not June 30?" I explained my reasoning and he agreed.

The meeting the following morning was the big monthly one in the boardroom where Snair would hand out awards to his buddies and attempt to turn the rest of us into quivering piles of raw nerve endings through the sheer cruelty of his words. This morning was mine, however. I called the shots today. I knew Snair was planning a caustic diatribe for me, but I was armed with the strongest counter-attack I would ever give him.

He started off, "Guess who missed quota, everybody?" He pointed at me and said very audibly and enthusiastically, glowing in my failure, "Jamie Blyth, come on down, son. Check out your prize." He then went off on one of his speeches, saying that failure could not be tolerated and there were repercussions for it. I was his exam-ple for half an hour. He predicted that I would miss quota this month and justly be fired, doing both the organization and myself a favor. If I missed one more month, it would mean that I wasn't any good and that I was in the wrong job anyway. That was the meeting when he told me I would eventually wind up in a nuthouse. "You laugh now," he said, "but when you're there, you'll look back in your white room and say, my God, he was right."

This man hadn't known what I had gone through in the last cou-ple of years, not that he would have cared. He glowed with power, mayhem, and lunacy. I let him continue, though, soaking it up, truly not letting him affect me for the first time in my life.

When Snair was done, I stood up and told him that I wanted the promotion today, on the day of my first failure. He said, "You're jok-ing, right? You're one month away from losing your job and you're asking for a promotion." I responded, "You told me to come to you when I wanted to challenge myself as a person and I am finally ready to do that."

He paused and stared me down for 10 seconds, thinking I would look away, but I didn't. Today, I was strong and game for anything he could throw at me. Today, I called the shots.

"All right. This will be fun," he said. "You realize your quota is going to be higher this month? This should be entertaining for me. Everybody, let's give Jamie a round of applause."

It was that easy, my paycheck stepped up along with my courage. I was going to beat this blowhard.

We went around in a circle and we gave Snair our projections of where we would be this month. I was last, on purpose. When it came to me, I threw down the biggest contract of my career. It was still only 8 a.m. on July 1 by this point. Gasps filled the room. Snair choked, "Are you telling me you sold that today?"

"Yes," I explained. "The guy was going to meet me yesterday, but he had a sick child at home. Instead, he agreed to see me before he left for vacation this morning. I met him at 6 a.m. for coffee."

Snair knew that I didn't drink coffee. I had him. For the first time, I had him stumped, speechless, at a complete loss.

I said, "My plan for this month is to work on my tan and play a lot of golf." It was great, because this gave me plenty of time to plan and build for the months ahead. By failing, I was ahead of the game, even though my record streak of hitting quota for 18 months in a row was over.

I was liberated. For the first time since the panic began, I felt totally empowered. Panic steals control from you, and those with panic attacks often desperately want to take back control of their lives. This little rebellion made me feel like I was in charge again. The panic couldn't dictate my future, and Snair couldn't bully or humiliate me into bending to his will.

This victory goes down in history as one of the most exhilarating moments of my life. I hadn't acted out of fear. I had done the thing I was most afraid of: I had failed, and I had let Snair trash me and point out all my weaknesses in front of the whole sales team. And at the end of it, I didn't want to go home and hide under the covers for days. In the end, I won.

■ ■ ■

It was perfect, and I admired him for it. If you're going to negotiate for position, you need to have a card to play. Most people lobby for positions when they don't deserve them. Jamie always deserved the opportunity because he was the best. He just never thought of himself as the best. I was probably harder on Jamie than I was on anyone in my career.

—Sam Snair (Jamie's old manager)

■ ■ ■

Sales served as a process of self-discovery for me. I realized I was good with people. I was (surprise!) a good speaker. Moreover, I was significant. I was worthy of happiness. I was not damaged goods. I had what it took to be successful, and I deserved success. Just knowing that gave me an emotional edge.

In his own twisted way, that's what Snair had been trying to pull out of me all along, and though we remained competitive with each other and traded jabs, we also formed an unlikely bond. He opened up to me about his troubled past, and I opened up to him about my anxiety disorder. It didn't make either of us pity each other, but maybe it made us respect each other some more and understand a bit more about what made one another tick.

When the pressures got to me, I'd often escape into great novels or lighthearted movies like *Caddyshack* or *Dumb and Dumber* to keep things in perspective. I called my funny friends—people who were positive and helped me lighten the load. Over time, I learned to thank God for all the blessings in my life instead of sulking about my obstacles. I even thanked him for that crazy antagonist Snair.

And then one day, after two and a half years with the company, the man just vanished. He cleared out his desk in the middle of the night and went to another firm. He'd entered my life like a tornado and left just as quickly, taking his buddies on the sales crew with him. I was immediately promoted to management after spending three years as a rep.

In his wake, I felt a release. The office seemed eerily quiet and calm. I felt a satisfying victory for having outlasted him, but the strangest thing happened in the months to follow: I started to miss the guy. I thought about him every day. I didn't get a chance to thank him for all he had taught me before he left.

My management days were priceless. I hadn't thought of myself as a leader since my grade school years, but here I was in charge of a sales force of 20 people, all of whom were older than I was. The new sales reps knew my reputation as a top earner, and they looked at me like an icon, a legend. They had no idea what it took to get me there.

Now I was the one standing in front of the room, with all eyes on me, training large groups of people on how to sell. It went a long way toward building my confidence.

Managers had to give monthly presentations to our corporate leaders, and most people relied on notes. I always overprepared and memorized my presentations. I wouldn't even have to look at the overhead projector to know which slide was showing; I'd already run through the presentation so many times in my head that I knew just the right moment to say, "Next slide, please." No matter how scared I was, I came across as confident and knowledgeable.

I went with the reps on sales calls and noticed how people who were nervous actually talked more. They felt the need to fill the uncomfortable silences with chatter, which didn't always work in their favor. I introduced my team to the same great reading material that had boosted me up—works by Viktor Frankl and Pat Riley—and asked them tough questions: What did they learn? How could they apply it to their lives? What were their dreams?

Just as I was counseling them, it occurred to me that I hadn't yet gone after many of my own dreams. Then the tragedy of September 11 happened and affected me the way it affected so many others—it forced me to reevaluate what I was doing to make mine a life worth living. I didn't want my tombstone to one day read, "Here lies a man who did great things for the telecommunications industry."

A building restlessness had been mounting inside of me and if I didn't do something about it quickly, my spirit would have died on me. I wanted to abandon my present existence and form a new path, start fresh.

I had gone as far as I could where I was. I met my goals and used this job as a way to build up my confidence, to find out who I was again. Once you've been through something extremely traumatic, like the anxiety disorder was to me, you never really return to being who you were before. If you're lucky, though, you get to be someone stronger. Better. And I wasn't going to get there while I was consumed with a world of quotas and expensive, pinchy shoes.

Social phobics like to stay in a routine, in a safe place. When we find a place that doesn't scare the wits out of us, we tend to stick around, and I knew I was in danger of getting stuck in the sales world because I was getting too comfortable with it. Safety, for me, diminishes growth, and I didn't feel like I was growing anymore. It was time to shake things up and create some discomfort.

So one night, I went into the barren office and wrote an e-mail to the staff. In part, it said:

> *"I went into the woods because I wished to live deliberately, to front only the essential facts of life, and see if I could not learn what it had to teach, and not when I came to die, discover that I had not lived."*
>
> **—Henry David Thoreau**

After much deliberation, I have decided to call it quits here. Last week's tragedy terrified the world and sickened us to the core, leaving us feeling vulnerable and lost and rearranged, forever altering the landscape of ourselves. After viewing the horrific images and hearing the countless stories of courage and selflessness, you can't help but view the world, your world, in a different light. Thoreau fittingly stated, "Not till we are lost, in other words not till we have lost the world, do we begin to find ourselves." There are some things I have always wanted to pursue and yet I never have. I just can't wait any longer.

I expected one or two responses. I got dozens—people saying that they understood and valued what I was doing and wanted to go after their passions too.

It wasn't a tough decision when I met Bob Muzikowski a couple of months later and he asked me to coach a Little League baseball team in the projects of Chicago. "I may not be able to solve the world's problems, but maybe I can encourage somebody to make the right choices," I told myself. Ninety percent of the kids in this Little League—the biggest inner-city program in the country, by the way—would wind up in jail at some point, if past statistics were still true. Maybe I couldn't erase that percentage, but if I could change one kid's future, it would be enough.

The movie *Hardball*, starring Keanu Reeves, was loosely based on Bob and his Little League accomplishments. Bob's life was spiraling out of control with alcohol and drug abuse, but he turned his life around through Alcoholics Anonymous and faith in God. A white businessman, he and his wife chose to move to the projects of Chicago and take a trashy field and turn it into a real Little League field. More than 200 kids signed up the first season. Bob had recruited local business people to help by donating money for uniforms, gloves, and bats—but he wouldn't let them just donate money. If they wanted to sponsor a team, he said, they had to coach it too. He wanted the kids to have good role models. Bob sees coaching as a ministry.

These kids don't get driven around in Acuras, they don't go to fancy dinners, and they'd never worry about getting some sales award for a trip to the Bahamas. They live in poverty-infested environments laden with drugs and stray bullets, and their heroes are rappers and gangsters. Only one kid on my team had a father at home. "I may not be the best person for the job, but it's a start," I thought. For myself and for them.

But I couldn't make a full-time career out of Little League coaching. When people asked me what I planned to do, I told them my three dreams: to play professional basketball, to be on television, and to write a book. I don't think any of them believed I would accomplish all that.

People stifled laughs when I told them I was going to play pro basketball. When I quit my job, I was in the worst shape of my life. I was more than 20 pounds overweight, and it wasn't muscle: it was chips and salsa, Budweiser, and pizza. But overcoming anxiety taught me to see a positive future, to see beyond my current limits. So I went straight to the gym, where a 45-year-old man beat the pants off me in one-on-one. Okay, I had a way to go.

My buddy Brian Musso, the former pro football player, agreed to train me. I asked him if he thought I could ever compete professionally, and he told me I was just as good as a lot of the pros, but I had never learned how to be an athlete. As Oprah would say, this was a lightbulb moment. If I could learn and unlearn panic, why couldn't I learn how to be an athlete?

The workouts were intense, and if you had seen my early runs, you would have laughed at me. If you put a book under my feet, I'm not sure I would have been able to jump over it. Musso focused on ingraining footwork and body positioning and movements so they'd eventually become automatic. Athletic training is largely teaching the brain to fire at the right moments. My neuromuscular responses had never been trained. I learned to love the feeling of pain in my legs and to fight through utter exhaustion, knowing that on the other side were growth and strength, a barrier broken through.

■ ■ ■

In their book *Painfully Shy,* the Markways observe the following:

Many studies have documented the benefits of aerobic exercise such as running, biking, swimming, or brisk walking. From a purely physical standpoint, the goal of aerobic exercise is to strengthen the cardiovascular system and increase stamina. From a psychological perspective, however, exercise can do much more. Research has demonstrated that 20 to 40 minutes of aerobic exercise leads to reduced anxiety and positive increases in mood, effects that last for several hours after the workout. Energy and concentration also receive a substantial boost from exercise. Perhaps most significant, a regular exercise program can enhance your general sense of well-being and quality of life.
—Barbara G. Markway, Ph.D., and Gregory Markway, Ph.D.

■ ■ ■

I implemented the same process that I had used to beat panic and to coach my Little League team: I focused on raising my self-esteem through preparation, hard work, a positive attitude, and easily attainable short-term goals that I would raise as my self-esteem improved.

If you're a manager in a car factory, you can't just sit and count cars, notice at the end of the day that there aren't enough, and yell at people to make more. You can't wait until the pressure is too much and then learn why you failed. It's too late by then. The process needs to be honed before that day begins. A basketball game may look like it's won with a three-point shot, but it's really won in a hot, empty gym in the summer when that player shot 500 times a day in preparation for that big moment.

At the end of our training, Musso admitted to me that I was the worst he had ever seen. He also said I made greater progress than anybody he had seen. It can help to gauge your performance with a benchmark. Mine was beating Musso—the best athlete I have ever seen—in one-on-one and just being able to play with my good friend Brian Wardle, who played pro ball and is still the second leading scorer in Marquette history. When I started, the members of my old high school team could slaughter me. Over the course of just a few months, this out-of-shape klutz was ready to become a pro point guard—the fastest position on the floor.

With that, I headed to Sweden.

Huh?

I wasn't even quite sure where Sweden was, and I had no plan whatsoever about where I would stay or how I would find a team once I got there. I had determined that I needed to go to Europe solely because pro basketball isn't as competitive there; in the United States, all we have is the NBA, and you have to be one of the best 300 players in the world to get on a team. I was realistic enough to know that wasn't going to happen.

My childhood friend Nathan Rowe had a girlfriend who was from Sweden, and she used to talk about how cool it was there. That's all it took. There really wasn't any other reason for me to go to Sweden rather than anywhere else in the world. It was about as calculated as throwing a dart at a map and deciding to fly to wherever the dart landed—maybe less so, because at least then I would have seen where the country was in relation to the United States. Faith conquered all, and I trusted that because I was following my true passion, good things would happen.

The end result wasn't as important as the growth and attitude that would develop. When you chase your dreams, you don't settle for mere existence. You push yourself as hard as you possibly can in the pursuit of excellence, and that leads to emotional growth. I wanted to live each day as if it were my last.

A television screen on the plane showed us the flight path with arrows. "Aha," I thought. "So *that's* where Sweden is." The plane landed in Stockholm, and a freezing rain pelted me as I tried to navigate my way through unfamiliar streets. I lived on a ship in the Baltic Sea for $10 a night—which included a midget's bed and a blanket arguably made of Saran Wrap—and spent my seasick days walking mile upon mile in search of pro basketball teams.

For a week, I surfed the Internet from cafés, contacted coaches, and walked from facility to facility in the hopes that someone, anyone, would give me a shot. It was like cold calling in sales. There, I had one month to make my quota. Now I had to accomplish a lifelong goal before my time ran out, and exhaustion wasn't going to stop me. Because I couldn't sleep on a rocking boat, I found places to catch naps. I was swiftly shown the door when a mattress store manager caught me snoring on a waterbed, and I was mistaken for a bum when I fell asleep in an art museum. My airline ticket was for only two weeks; now I had just seven days to find a team with an opening for a point guard. Feeling desperate, I asked every random stranger I saw—people at Burger Kings and CD shops, businessmen walking down the street—if they knew where I could find a pro hoops team in Sweden.

■ ■ ■

From: "Brian Loftus"
To: "Jamie Blyth"
Subject: Keep Trying!
Date: Fri, 8 Feb 2002

Jamie,

Sounds difficult, interesting, invigorating, and very Blyth-like thus far. I knew it wouldn't be easy. Don't get down on yourself if it doesn't happen during the course of this trip.

You can always go back. It sounds like a lot of logistics . . . seems almost like you're chasing your tail at times, but, remember, one impressive performance on the court where you outplay solidified team members could go a long way.

You still have 10 days. Kurt Cobain was homeless the day "Nevermind" was released in 1991. Brad Pitt was delivering refrigerators to homeowners when he landed *A River Runs Through It*. Paul Pierce was dodging bullets on the worst courts in L.A. when Kansas offered him a scholarship. A life-changing, positive result can come out of your efforts. The physical, mental, and emotional challenge you're experiencing can be translated into a pro contract with some solid play on the court.

Don't put pressure on yourself, just get out on the court and play your game.

■ ■ ■

Ninety-nine percent of those I asked looked at me like I had an ear growing out of my forehead, though they were friendly and wanted to be helpful. Things looked bleak until I walked into a Footlocker and struck up a conversation with a salesman who told me how to get to the practice facility of the top team in Sweden.

On the train ride there, I collected my thoughts about how I'd "sell myself" to the general manager. "Well, Kevin, I never played college hoops, I've actually been in technology sales and management for four years, and my golf game is steadily improving." As it turned out, Kevin Ryan was the perfect person to run into: he was a Canadian living his dream, and he wanted to give me the chance to live mine.

"You've come this far," he said. "I'll give you four days to make it or break it. Practice starts at 11:30 a.m. tomorrow. Here's a ball if you want to get some shots up. Good luck!"

■ ■ ■

Jamie can just go overseas, not know where these basketball teams are playing, not communicate with a single person beforehand, can get off an airplane and go to a sports store and say, "Hey, where's the basketball team?" The crazy thing about Jamie and the marvelous thing is that to him, that's not strange. And I think it was the best thing he ever could have done.

—Nathan Rowe

■ ■ ■

Exhausted from jetlag and walking the length of the whole darn country with huge bags strapped to my chest and back and suffering from a sore throat that made it feel like I was trying to swallow a brick, I didn't exactly dazzle them for the first three days. I vomited at the end of the first practice, and players laughed at me as I was crouched over, ragged, beaten down before even the warm-ups ended. But I never quit. "Five minutes longer," I kept telling myself. "Hang in there five minutes longer."

Then came the miraculous fourth day where everything came together. I was in the zone and the basket was as big as a quarry as I made every shot in sight—fade away jump shots, reverse layups, three-pointers. I owned that court. My defenders seemed like a blur as I flew past them effortlessly to the basket.

I walked home in the frigid night, giddy and amazed at what had just happened. When I think of that night under the Stockholm stars, a warm nostalgia floods me, memories of struggle and wonder, belief and joy. I stopped on the bridge over the Baltic Sea, taking it all in. Far across the shimmering moonlit water, I saw an unidentified blinking light, blinking as if just for me, like I was the only one who could see it. I thought of the many years since my first panic attack and how far I had traveled, seemingly the length of my soul. I thought of those years locked in fear and despair, when I was unable to see the light of hope that burned through the cold, shadowy darkness. And I smiled.

I made the team.

·· 12 ··

Carpe Diem

Victory belongs to the most persevering.
—NAPOLEON

Much as it pained me to have to give up that midget bed and the blanket the size of a Wet Nap, I deigned to accept my new team-mate's parents' offer to let me stay in their home. We ate delicious Swedish pancakes for dinner, a Tuesday tradition for them, and laughed into the wee hours of the night. (The pizza, on the other hand, was a disaster.) I couldn't believe they were trusting a swarthy stranger like me to stay in their guest bedroom.

"You'd do the same for us if we were in America, right?" Mr. Hedstrom asked.

Just like that, my living conditions improved from a dismal room at sea to one of the nicest condos in Stockholm. I didn't even feel a hint of anxiety around these people, which shocked me.

Swedes are a unique breed. They're open and friendly and a bit quirky. They say "of course" an inordinate amount. During a five-minute conversation, a Swede will say "of course" at least 10 times, and that's par for the course . . . of course. Around them, I felt loose and free—human, even.

I experienced things more and got to know people better because I was able to live in the present and hear and feel what was going on around me. Panic blocks these emotions and clouds any chance for true experience. The enormous amount of self-consciousness and worry becomes the focal point: Will I lose control? My heart is beating too fast. I feel weak and off-balance . . . am I going to panic in front of these people? But now, none of those fears invaded my thoughts, and I was able to be myself on and off the court.

I felt as though I had cleared some barrier within myself—like the fog I had wandered through for too many years had lifted and allowed me to see clearly again. There was no safety net, and the only "escape" would be an international plane ride, and yet that was fine by me. This experience in Sweden would give me an edge and I knew it. If I ever felt panic coming back, I could point to this experience and use it to ignite me and remind me that I had the potential to be at ease, even in unfamiliar territory.

After I had lived in their house for only a few days, the Hedstroms asked me to watch their house while they went skiing in the Alps for a week and a half. "This would never happen in America," I told myself. What trust they had in me!

All I had to do was feed the turtles in their aquarium. Great deal! Unfortunately—and here's the reason why I hope the Hedstroms never read this book—it *may* be possible that I *might* have forgotten to do even that for a few days, and it's *possible* that I nearly killed those poor turtles.

About six weeks later, I was on the subway coming home from practice and having a conversation with an older Swedish couple when a group of about six Turkish teenagers caught on that I was American and decided to harass me.

"I love Osama Bin Laden!" the group's "leader" proclaimed. This was February of 2002, the wounds of September 11 still fresh in my mind. Although disturbed, I tried to ignore him and continued my conversation with the couple. The kid said it again, though, louder this time to make sure I heard him clearly. I asked him to keep his opinions to himself, but he said, "This is not America. You're in Sweden and I can say whatever I want. I love Osama Bin Laden!"

"You're right, you can say whatever you want," I said. "Just know that the next time you say it, you will not have any teeth left."

I felt like Clint Eastwood—like Dirty Harry in Sweden.

"There are six of us and one of you," the kid said.

"True, but your teeth will still be gone. I'm not going after them, I'm going after you. You guys may win, but I will get you. Your choice. I suggest you choose wisely."

He looked at me and smiled. I stood up.

"You have 10 seconds to wipe that smile off your face and then I want you to apologize. I knew people who died in those buildings." I lasered in on his eyes and began counting aloud. People stared at me with mouths agape, eyes widening at the display that was unfolding before them. "10, 9, 8, 7 . . ." When I got to 3, the kid gulped and apologized, then got off the train at the next stop.

Where had that courage come from? When had I learned how to stand up for myself like that? There hadn't been a trace of fear, and although I later wasn't proud of myself for threatening violence, I was still proud of myself for not being a doormat. Score one for the social phobic.

When I got back to the United States in March, I returned with a fortified spirit and fantastic sense of accomplishment. People asked about my job, and I said, "I'm a point guard. I play basketball." I couldn't believe I was actually saying those words, but it was true. What was perhaps cooler was that it didn't seem to surprise anyone; it was now part of who I was, who I always should have been.

In serious need of warm weather, I cashed in an unused trip I had won from my sales job and headed to L.A. to see Brian Loftus and his new girlfriend, Jenny. We went to dinner at the famous Rainbow

Room, and halfway through the meal, Jenny told me she thought I'd be great for the show where she was working as an assistant producer: *The Bachelor*. I asked her what kind of show it was and she looked at me cock-eyed, as if she was waiting for me to tell her I was kidding.

"You've never seen it?" she asked when she realized I was serious. "It's a dating show with 1 guy and 25 girls. The Bachelor narrows the field down by going on a series of dates with the hope of finding true love and marriage. You would be the star of the show for the second season."

Brian thought it was a great idea. He told me it would give him plenty of entertainment, watching me make an idiot of myself every week on television.

Without thinking much, and running on sheer adrenaline and fantasy, I said, "Cool! What do I need to do?"

She told me I'd have to send the producers a tape of myself, and I agreed to do it. But as I thought about it, I realized that this was reality TV. You can't prepare for that. It's living without a net and in front of the whole world. And besides, it's a dating show! I got nervous dating just one girl—how could I date 25 of them on national television?

The thought kept pinballing around in my mind as I argued with myself. One part of me thought it would be a blast, and the other thought it was way too much pressure. Why mess with the positive mindset I had developed? I was feeling pretty safe and comfortable in the world; why should I throw myself into a situation that could reignite my panic?

Back in Chicago, I talked to friends about it. Joe and his new wife Alexis freaked out when I asked them what they thought. "Are you kidding me?" Alexis screamed. "I love that show! You need to do that tape!"

There was a deadline for turning in the tape, and I was three weeks late. Procrastinating. Finally, I handed my mom a video camera and told her to interview me. We stood outside her house, and for 10 minutes, my mom asked me relationship questions that made me feel pretty awkward. What physical qualities attract me to a girl? (Symmetrical ears.) What did I like to do on dates? (Play checkers.) Why am I a good catch? (I usually remember to put the toilet seat down.)

Seriously, I have no idea what I said. I never watched it. Sometimes I'd mess up and rewind a little, unable to see what was happening on the tape, and just take a guess at where I'd left off and tell my mom to keep going.

That tape sat on my dresser for weeks while I agonized about whether or not to send it in. Maybe I put it off so it would be too late and then I'd say, "Darn! I would have done it if only I hadn't missed the deadline." A giant *if* played in my mind—I might be able to handle it . . . *if* my anxiety remained dormant. I didn't know if I could count on that.

Fear is what held me back, and that's exactly what spurred me to send it in.

Avoidance is death. Fear wasn't going to hold me back anymore. This was going to be the ultimate way to challenge my fears and prove to myself once and for all that I could handle anything that life threw my way.

So just before I boarded a plane to Germany for a two-week basketball camp, I handed my mom that tape and told her to take it to the post office for me. Once it was out of my hands, the tension lifted: it was no longer something I could control. Now it was up to producers to decide whether or not I'd face my fears on national TV.

I, on the other hand, landed in Frankfurt and was to hop on a train to Cologne, the location of a camp where scouts and coaches would evaluate pro-level talent from 36 countries. With my success in Sweden, I now had a small résumé and a reason for other pro teams to take me seriously.

Waiting for the train, I caught a glimpse of a beautiful girl sitting on her suitcase. I walked by her to get a better look and was mesmerized by her hazel-green eyes and flowing brown hair. Our eyes met and I needed an excuse to talk to her, quick!

"Hi. Do you know which track the train to Cologne is going to be on?" I asked.

"I'm not sure either," she said, "but that's my train too."

Sabina was her name. We found the train, and I helped her with her heavy bag. She followed me into my compartment, where we talked the whole two-hour trip, rolling along the beautiful Rhine River and the green hills and vineyards. She had a sweet voice and demeanor, and we weren't ready to part when the train came to a stop. We headed to a café, and while we stared up at the most impressive cathedral I've ever seen, she told me she thought something big was about to happen in my life, but she didn't know what.

I found love—or at least quick affection—for a girl on a train in Germany. Maybe that social anxiety was really behind me after all.

We met daily and nightly for coffee and wine. By then, I had recklessly started drinking the real stuff (caffeine) again. I wanted to feel like anybody else and quit curtailing my pleasures because of this lousy disorder.

Sabina poured her heart out to me, and I told her that I might go to Hollywood and write a book someday. I fantasized about getting a basketball contract in Germany and staying there and marrying her—this girl I'd known for a week.

On the second day of scrimmages, I played so well that a German coach walked up to me at the end and we were negotiating a contract within 10 minutes. He asked me where I had gone to school. "Illinois," I told him. "We were a top 25 team." Well, we were. He didn't have to know that I wasn't actually *on* the team, right? I told him about Stockholm and handed him a tape of scrimmages I'd done in a pick-up game with college friends who were solid players.

Confidently, I let him know that I expected the standard housing, car, and salary. I had no idea what kind of salary he had in mind, but I tried to look like I'd done this a million times before. He offered a small salary plus a car and housing for a nine-month contract. I told him I had a team in Sweden who'd offered me more, and that I'd sign with him if he gave me an extra 10 grand. He agreed, and said he just wanted to look at my tape before finalizing the deal.

Later, I checked my e-mail at an Internet café and found a letter from ABC, telling me I was one of eight finalists for *The Bachelor*. They wanted me to fly straight to L.A. when I left Germany the following week. My heart pounded—this time in a good way. I forwarded the e-mail to friends and family and mused about this fast-paced fantasy I was living.

I checked myself in the mirror—I had taken a charge and an elbow from a Russian player and had nine stitches under my right eye, so the face they saw on the tape was a bit mangled. "Maybe they like the rugged look," I thought.

Before I went to L.A., though, they had to put me under a microscope. I filled out a 30-page questionnaire and went for drug and STD tests. They called 10 references outside of my family and drilled them about my life and character. My brother told me it was the kind of background check the FBI would do. I left Germany buzzing with possibility and energy—I had a solid opportunity to play ball in Germany, I'd met a great girl, and I could possibly star in a TV show.

I had built these ABC people up in my mind to be larger than life. My Midwestern mind thought of these manicured Hollywood executives in power suits and wondered if I could ever live up to the movie star mystique they were used to. I was just a regular guy who liked to play hoops and hang out with my friends. But I landed in

L.A. with enthusiasm and hope, and above all, a great sense of adventure.

A man in dark sunglasses who looked suspiciously like Will Smith's character from *Men in Black* met me at the airport, and he was holding a sign that said "Tom Slater." That was to be my alias so the press didn't catch on to who the next Bachelor might be. I walked over to this gentleman, laughing at the absurdity of the situation.

"Hi, I'm Slater . . . Tom Slater," I said.

Blam! Two cameras were thrust inches away from my face before the man could respond. I couldn't have been taken more off-guard if Halle Berry had walked by and offered to carry my bags.

Producers and film crew from the show followed me around the airport with their cameras rolling, instructing me to act natural and not look at the cameras. I wheeled around with shocked eyes, telling myself to act cool and unaffected. I actually did act like myself—I got lost trying to find my bags and stumbled around aimlessly for 15 minutes until I found the right baggage claim. "Great job, Jamie," I thought. "Do what you would normally do . . . get lost."

Acting unaffected is pretty tough when every single move you make is being recorded so that producers can pore through the footage later and scrutinize your facial expressions and your posture. People stared at me as I walked through the airport and out to the limo. They thought I was a celebrity. I was too much in shock to panic.

Once we got to the studio, the first interview commenced. My first performance was dull and expressionless. I knew it, but I was stuck in survival mode at that point—just trying to hang on and suppress my anxiety in front of the camera. I didn't have time to settle in, and I was frustrated that I had no idea how to prepare for something like this.

A producer named Haley was playful with me and trying to pump me up. "Come on, Jamie, this is your big shot. Make it happen."

When my stage presence remained that of a slug's, she asked the camera guy to turn the camera on her instead. She instructed me to ask her questions, and she demonstrated the bubbly enthusiasm that she wanted me to emulate.

I turned into a slug on sleeping pills instead. As soon as the camera was off, I felt my fear subside. This was just the beginning, I knew, and even though I hadn't impressed anybody yet, I had survived phase one.

Next came a psychological evaluation. "Ha! Just what I need," I thought. Thank God the cameras left me alone for this part of the process.

"Do you kill animals?" the test asked. "Nope," I confidently checked. They had a bunch of these sorts of questions to make sure they didn't have an axe murderer on their hands. Then they had several questions relating to anxiety, depression, and emotional instability. I lied my butt off.

Afterward, I spoke to their psychologist and felt perfectly comfortable around her. I gave a rousing and convincing performance. When she asked if I'd ever felt emotionally out of control or contemplated suicide, I said, "No way. Life's too good." Part of me wanted to tell her how I was really feeling, but I knew that would ruin my chances. I later found out that she had picked me as her top choice to do the show.

When I met Haley in the hall later, I extended an enthusiastic, "Hey, what's up?"

"How did the meeting go?" she asked.

"Great. I am certifiably nuts and I lied through my teeth and she bought it."

I exuded confidence and enthusiasm, riding this roller coaster of emotions and strength, just the way she wished I was on camera. Haley told me that cameras would barge in on me anytime over the next few days and I'd do random interviews, starting with the producers and working my way up to the head honchos of the show and the network. "Perfect!" I said, hoping she wouldn't notice I was scared to death.

In my room, I did breathing exercises and read positive affirmations and quotes from my notebook. Then I went outside and ran sprints until I nearly collapsed. I always seem to gain something from physical exhaustion that comes from exercise, from pushing myself as hard as I can and just when I'm about to give up, pushing a little more. It fortifies and relaxes me.

Producers burst into my room every couple of hours and asked me questions to see how I would react to the frequent "surprises." My head was spinning when it finally hit the pillow around 2 a.m. My call time was 7:00 the next morning. I wasn't allowed to leave my room or call anybody, except when I got permission to go out and exercise. But my buddy Brian managed to sneak a quick call through by dialing the hotel and asking for Tom Slater!

At 6 a.m., I was awakened by my annoying alarm clock and an intrepid cameraman. He waited for me, and when I was remotely decent—meaning that I had a towel around my waist—he filmed me brushing my teeth, shaving, and changing. Boy, that was weird. Never before had I considered whether or not my toothbrushing habits were film-worthy. I just prayed I didn't dribble any paste down my chin. I guessed I was going to have to get used to this.

We walked down to a hotel room where there was a chair planted in the middle, surrounded by cameras, white backdrops, and bright spotlights. Across from me was a row of chairs. The crew instructed me to sit down and they miked me, something that's old hat to me now. The mike goes under your shirt and then is clipped or taped just out of sight on the collar. They offered me water, and I tried to control the desperation in my voice as I accepted and cleared my throat far too many times.

I felt like a lab rat as they positioned the cameras and lights to be as invasive of my personal space as possible. The producers gave me brief training about how to answer questions. The key was to make it appear as if I were not being asked questions, but merely talking. If they asked me "Why should you be our next Bachelor?" I would have to repeat the question to pinpoint the context, then respond, "I would make a good Bachelor because . . . blah, blah, blah."

I held up fine during these interviews, but I did not thrive. I just wasn't comfortable enough to bring out my optimum self. In this strange and overwhelming environment, my personality and humor got lost. The producers were friendly, and I could tell they were pulling for me—especially Lisa, who told everybody that I should be given a chance based on that tape my mom sent in. I could tell I was letting her down during the interview, that I wasn't the person she hoped I would be. Her face pleaded with me to liven up.

I was pleased with myself for getting through this, but mad at myself for not being able to "bring it on." After the interview, I felt Snair on my shoulder, challenging me to bring out the basketball player that always rested somewhere within.

Down in the lobby, when I went to catch a late dinner, I ran into Lisa sitting on a couch having drinks with the director and creator of the show. I said "Hi," and they invited me to sit down and chat. I told them that I was nervous.

■ ■ ■

I remember everybody around was teasing me because I was so smitten with him I couldn't even conduct the interview. I thought he was just *so* gorgeous. But when he sat down, he was sort of quiet and nonresponsive and very uncomfortable. He was just not himself. I ran into him later in the lobby, and I had a beer with him. And he was the greatest guy ever. That's when he said, "Listen, I'm sorry, I blew it. I just really froze." . . . stuff like that.

And I said, "You know what, Jamie, that's okay. I think you're a little too young to be The Bachelor anyway; you've got more of your life ahead of you. When things come up, maybe we'll get together again. I have lots of shows."

—Lisa Levenson, executive producer, ABC

■ ■ ■

We talked for about five minutes and my tension faded. For the first time, these people were seeing my true colors, and I was determined to make it last over the next two days.

I did improve in front of the cameras, but I was inconsistent. They tried to trip me up to see how well I could handle pressure: "You are going to have 25 women. How are you going to narrow the field down? You don't believe in love at first sight? Then how are you going to make a decision in one night and cut 10 women? That doesn't make sense. Are you sure you mean that? How are you going to handle the scrutiny of the cameras and get engaged at the end of six weeks? Prove it."

They were tough, but in the end, I knew I did a good job and earned that sale and had them back on my side. At the end of that third day, some people had me as their number 1 choice, others as their number 2. But on my last day, something occurred to me: I could really *get* this gig. Do I really *want* this gig?

Did I want to get married on national TV? Was I even ready for marriage, let alone with someone I would only know for six weeks? "Be careful what you wish for, because you just may get it," I thought. And consequently, my final interview just wasn't as fiery. The doubts in my mind were logical this time, not just based on my anxiety disorder.

After that last interview, the staff wished me a good flight home and told me they'd be in touch. They sounded like me after I interviewed someone I knew I wasn't going to hire.

I savored my last glimpse of the world of television and Hollywood, and I left with a unique experience. There are worse disappointments in life than not being The Bachelor, right? I couldn't be too hard on myself; I had taken on a wildly high-pressure situation, and even if I wasn't perfect, I held up just fine. Besides, in August, I was going to play pro hoops in Germany.

But a few months later, Lisa called me and told me about this new show they were doing where the situation would be reversed: 25 men and 1 woman. The pressure wouldn't all be on the man this time.

"Would you like to be on *The Bachelorette*?" she asked.

Life on Film

When you cannot make up your mind
which of two evenly balanced courses of action
you should take . . . choose the bolder.
—EZRA POUND

By choosing *The Bachelorette*, I knew I was probably wiping out my chances of ever playing pro hoops in Germany again. I had to turn the coach down and tell him I'd be out of commission for the next year because of the show and its aftermath. Both of my dreams were converging at once and I had to make this heart-wrenching—but cool—decision. I had already proven to myself that I could handle playing basketball, but going on reality TV? This was the ultimate way to test myself.

Social phobics have an intense fear of situations that could cause humiliation, rejection, judgment, or discomfort in front of people. The concept of this show would challenge every one of those fears. And I could hardly wait.

"Who knows?" I thought. "I could even meet the girl of my dreams." It seemed unlikely, but I had learned by now that nothing was impossible. What I lost in my race to defeat panic and depression and to be the top sales guy was love. My life had a laser beam, single-minded focus, and so much energy had gone into this area that I had left the romantic part of my life vacant. From ages 19 to 24, I probably went on two dates. Over the past two years, I had begun dating again, but I have to admit that I was feeling pretty lonely and didn't mind the possibility of finding a woman to whom I could give myself fully.

I think I expected the anxiety to grab hold of me in those months before *The Bachelorette*, but really, it didn't. I had a normal amount of nervousness in the week before I had to leave, but it didn't consume me. I had finally realized that I was significant as a person—that I measured up and had worth. My punishing thoughts and "what ifs" were shed like an old skin, and I focused on preparing myself for the task at hand as best as I could.

On the prowl for ways to get used to the feeling of being on display, I went to karaoke bars and sang my heart out. (By the way, I'm a lousy singer.) At weddings or clubs, I was the first person out on the dance floor, sometimes the only person. (Oh, and I dance with the rhythm of a turkey.)

My friends had a blast because I let them choose the songs I'd sing in karaoke and they got to watch me flail around on the dance floor. Then I'd barge into a table full of girls, initiate conversation, and ask one of them if she would go out with me. If she said no, I'd go down the line until one agreed or they all said no. It was humiliating, but I wanted to put myself in as many uncomfortable situations as possible to prepare for my television performance.

My friends Brian Loftus and Brian Musso gave me encouraging pep talks as my departure date got closer. When I left for the show, I did so with a feeling that I had done all I could, and now whatever was going to happen would happen. It was going to be okay no matter what.

My fellow Bachelors and I were sequestered in a hotel for a few days before the show began, and we weren't allowed to make phone calls or talk to anyone who might be involved with the show. If we wanted to leave the hotel, we had to get permission from our "watcher." I went a little stir-crazy during these days and it gave my anxiety plenty of time to play tricks on me. I did all my relaxation techniques, but I knew that I was just going to have to face this situation head-on. The night before filming began, I went out to an unoccupied parking lot in Universal Studios and ran sprints, exhausting myself.

It turns out that Ryan, another Bachelor from the show, whom I hadn't met yet, was watching me from his window. He has told me that he was moments away from joining me when I walked away. Later, I'd find out what a great athlete he was—he played college football and even made it to the NFL and played for the Carolina Panthers. Unfortunately, he tore his shoulder apart on his very first play and never played again. We hit it off instantly because of our mutual love for sport.

My basketball buddies had coached me on how to greet Trista, The Bachelorette. Brian Wardle told me to play it cool and not do anything over-the-top, my ex-coaches suggested I give her a rose, and another buddy told me to slap her on the butt as I walked by. In the end, I opted to be myself and greet her with a simple introduction.

Anxiety did visit me in the beginning of the show. In fact, I briefly considered going home because I wasn't sure I could hack it. "This is a character-building experience," I reminded myself. "You knew what you were getting into, and you wanted to feel this fear."

If I was going to find out what I was made of, I would have to bear it. I'd have to go through the fear and complete the experience, no matter how it turned out. After I got to California, I had second thoughts about whether or not I was really ready for this or whether it might jeopardize my recovery if it didn't turn out well. But I'm so glad I stuck around—it wound up being the best experience of my life.

The first night, all 25 guys and Trista got to meet and talk for the first time, and if you didn't know better, you probably would have thought that I was the most confident guy in the room. I went around the whole room asking everyone questions about themselves, making wisecracks, and getting everyone laughing. The producers even told me to quit being the host of the show.

Each week culminated in a "rose ceremony." This was where Trista chose who would stay another week and who would be eliminated. She did this by handing a rose to each of the men she was inviting to stay. Anyone left without a rose had an awkward minute to say goodbye, then leave the show. The rose ceremonies began at around 7 p.m. and typically went on until 5 or 6 a.m. Trista had to talk to each man individually for about 15 to 20 minutes apiece, and the filming process itself is long and tedious. Sound has to be tested, lights have to be set and reset, camera angles adjusted. Suffice it to say I was pretty exhausted by the time I received my roses!

During the first rose ceremony, nerves were definitely firing all around. Bob cut the tension with his ridiculous Irish jig dance, then followed it up by belting out Journey tunes. We all laughed and started goofing off to the point where the director had to settle us down and get us back to business.

My fear of rejection was not so focused on Trista as it was on missing the rest of the experience. If she cut me this soon, I'd have to go home. I figured out right away that I wasn't going to marry this woman, but ABC does a great job of building up tension, both for the participants and for the audience. Who would stay? Who would go? It was an agonizing wait, but each time I got to stick around, I was thrilled.

■ ■ ■

My first impression of Jamie was basically, "Damn it! I love the kid!" All I could think, really, was that he's such a good-looking guy and he's got such a great personality that he is a shoo-in. And then to have a great jump shot on top of that? I'm going home!

—Bob Guiney (competitor on *The Bachelorette*)

■ ■ ■

Sleep was not an option at *The Bachelorette* house. There were lights and cameras on us for all but about two hours a day, and even if I wanted to sleep under blinding lights, people like Bob and Charlie (two other contestants) made it clear that rest would not be tolerated. I managed to sneak about two hours of sleep a night, but that was it. We stayed up late getting to know each other, and I quickly realized that these were not the slick, sleazy Hollywood guys I would have expected to be on a show like this. The truth—and I'm not saying this to be polite—is that we got along fantastically and I made many lasting friendships with the other Bachelors, the host, and the crew.

I was able to be myself again. Unlike the years of panic when all of my attention was focused on my symptoms and hiding them, here I was able to stop monitoring myself enough so that I was able to really pay attention to other people. In the group setting, my anxiety fell and fell as I got to know the guys better and feel comfortable around them.

We spent nights playing pool, laughing, telling all of our stories. Greg had a guitar, and Bob is a good singer, so they often played and we'd all listen or sing along. The production staff scolded us with regularity because we were belting out songs while they were trying to conduct interviews. They couldn't show us singing these songs because the songs were copyrighted, they explained, so we started making up our own songs. One was called "Pony Chow."

People always ask me what I was thinking on the night that I dumped the dog food over my head. It's a convoluted story, but I'll do my best to tell it. About a week after the show started, the producers came up to Bob and me and said, "You two are always goofing around. Ryan is writing poems, Greg is writing songs, Russ bought a Tiffany bracelet . . . what are you doing for Trista?"

"I bought her a pony on eBay," Bob deadpanned. "It'll be waiting for her after the show, but we'd better hurry, because it's on its last hoof. His name is Gluestick."

I, of course, was laughing, and when they asked me what I was doing for her, I said, "I bought her half a sack of Pony Chow for Gluestick."

The other guys heard about this and they created a song based on the story. Easily half of Bob's conversations with Trista revolved around this horse that didn't exist. She thought we were nuts, I think, but she had a great sense of humor.

We had a dog on the show, and, as you may recall, Greg had a special affinity for Goldie. When Bob was beat out by Greg, producers asked how he felt about Greg's going further and he said, "I thought the only blonde Greg was interested in was Goldie!" Because we couldn't show brand names on TV, we had relabeled the dog food Pony Chow instead of Puppy Chow.

For some reason, Bob had thrown the bag of dog food on the roof and it spilled everywhere. He went up to the roof to sweep it off, and that's when Trista arrived after a date with Greg. "What are you doing sweeping dog food off the roof?" she asked, quite sensibly. She didn't stay long.

I can't explain this next part any better than the fact that being cooped up without any TV, reading material, radio, or contact with the outside world, coupled with the constant pressure of video cameras scrutinizing your every move, creates an environment of lunacy. That night, we had all been partying pretty hard and everybody chanted "Pony Chow!" I came out and dumped the bag over my head.

That was me proving to myself that I didn't care what anyone thought of me, not even the gazillions of viewers who were now going to wonder about my sanity. That was me realizing that my self-worth was no longer going to be determined by how well I could put on a false front and try to "impress" people. I was so relaxed by this point in the show that I was able to cut loose in front of the guys and quit worrying about what the cameras might or might not pick up on.

■ ■ ■

He does a good job of masking his anxiety. He would be extremely goofy, like when he did the thing with the dog food. It's so overboard that no one would ever think this guy has a problem hanging out with people, because he seems so comfortable being so silly in front of people.

—Ryan Sutter (winner of *The Bachelorette*)

■ ■ ■

The following day was a group date to Palm Springs with Bob, Ryan, Jack, Brian, and me. The ride there was the best time I had on the show. They didn't air it on the program, but Gluestick and our bachelor pad antics became the topic of conversation for the whole ride. Bob and I broke into our Abbott and Costello–like routine. Trista cried with laughter the whole trip and later said it was the best group date she went on. I felt totally at ease and was having a great time.

In fact, I *always* felt at ease unless I was alone with Trista. I beat the others in "Rock, Paper, Scissors" to score a one-on-one date, and we went to get massages. We sat on two beds and made chitchat while two women massaged our backs. My face was only a foot away from Trista's, and there were probably 30 people watching and two cameras directly in my face. It was unnerving, to say the least, and I wondered if the microphone would pick up my heart beating.

"Your back is very tight," the masseuse said. "You must be under a lot of stress."

You think so? Thirty million people are about to watch me getting a massage while on a first date with a beautiful woman. What could possibly be stressful about that?

Trista asked me about my family and I responded, "I have a mom and dad, brother . . . two brothers . . . and a younger sister." Quite the conversationalist, no? It was like I was trying to conserve words so I didn't run out of them later.

I knew Trista must have seen my sudden shift in personality. I was so extroverted in the group setting, but one-on-one, I tend to be quieter unless I know the person well. Now the pressure and attention was all on me, which made me feel more subdued and nervous. It was really my first long encounter alone with her and I did fine, but I didn't show the flashy, outgoing personality I had shown before.

■ ■ ■

On our first group date on the show on the way to a spa, we were on a bus, like a rock 'n' roll bus. Jamie was just having a good ol' time with all the guys. Of course, later on he just seemed a little more out of his element when he was with me by myself. Obviously, there were cameras around, so it could have been the fact that there were cameras. But he was definitely a little bit more nervous. I just thought he had low self-confidence.

—Trista Rehn Sutter (The Bachelorette)

■ ■ ■

The producers got us up and I felt relieved. Not an extraordinary job, but I'd made it through the date unscathed.

Then the producers told us the second part of the date would be in the shower. Say *what*? They led us to one of those showers where the water kind of pours out everywhere. Granted, I had basketball shorts on and she had a beautiful blue bikini, but my head pretty much exploded. "I'm in a shower on a first date . . . with some girl I don't even know . . . what the heck am I supposed to do?"

My heart pounded wildly and I felt sort of shell-shocked and confused. "My mom is watching," I thought. "And have I mentioned I'm in a *shower* with some *girl I don't know*?"

Act natural. Act natural. Pretend you're in your bathroom at home and no one is watching. I literally just started to take a shower

. . . washing my hair, my underarms . . . then Trista tapped on my back and said, "You have company."

Oh yeah. Forgot. Do I kiss her? No, I don't even know her. What can I do?

I saw the suds and was saved: I could wash her back! I stood there lathering up her back with my arms extended like a freak robot. Very awkward, but some people actually said it looked sensual. Ah, the power of editing.

Back at the bachelor pad, I told the guys about what had happened and we had a great laugh. We were not competitive with one another; we were all just enjoying the experience and becoming friends. They were down-to-earth guys and, in the end, we all wanted the winner to be whoever had the best connection with Trista.

■ ■ ■

Everyone certainly went into it just being themselves and kind of hoping for the best, I think. But the best didn't necessarily mean that they were going to be the ones to end up with Trista. It was the same way with me. I just happened to be the one who lucked out in the end. But I never felt like I needed to one-up somebody or I needed to sell somebody out or anything like that. I think everyone felt the same way. I think that's why we're all such good friends—we were totally up-front and honest with each other and didn't try to backstab or be dishonest.

—Ryan Sutter

■ ■ ■

Ryan had smuggled in Thoreau's *Walden*—one of my favorite books, despite the fact that it was what I was reading when I had my first panic attack—and we spent hours talking about the symbolism and what Thoreau must have meant. (I can't imagine why they didn't air our great philosophies!) So it didn't surprise me much when, during the second week, I walked in to talk to Ryan and he was writing a poem.

"That's cool, man," I said. "I used to write poems every now and then. Do you mind telling me what it's about?"

"It's a love poem to Trista."

I spit out my drink. When I told Bob, he jokingly said, "Okay, we can't talk to him anymore. He's way more into this than we are. Let's go play a round of Blackjack."

Now, don't get me wrong—I thought Trista was great. Really cute and sweet. But Ryan was already using the "L" word and I was still trying to remember that her name was Trista, not Trisha. That was probably my first faux pas: One of the first times I met her, I asked, "Trisha, do you like golf?" She answered, "My name is Trista and I hate golf." Bob and Charlie overheard and wouldn't let me live it down. Every time they got a chance, they'd walk up to her and ask, "Trisha, do you like golf?"

I swear I've never laughed as much as I did during that show. What they show on the air can make everybody seem one-dimensional, and it's not always accurate. It was clear that they had certain qualities they wanted to show in each of us—Russ was the crazy and aggressive guy, Charlie was the smooth and polished Casanova, Bob was the funny guy, Ryan was the sensitive poet, and I was the Ken doll shy guy.

But if you asked the others, they would have said that I was outgoing and wild and funny. Ryan jokingly called me Captain America. I think they all expected me to go down to the wire with Trista (so did the odds-makers—at the end of the first show, Vegas had me winning by 94 percent). Of course, the guys never saw the few encounters when I was alone with Trista and I was more reserved. When the show aired, Charlie said it was cool to see that side of me. He thought I was always the outlandish, outgoing type.

Charlie came off as very serious on the show, but in truth, he has a biting sense of humor; he's really sarcastic and funny. I wasn't expecting Russ to come off as intense about Trista as he appeared, either. And Ryan wasn't *always* writing poetry. He's quiet in a group setting, but was very talkative with me. Ryan talks when he really has something to say.

Even though they were at odds on the show, Charlie and Russ wound up being close friends afterward. "I know I called him a jerk," Charlie said, "but he's the nicest guy once you get past that 'Type A' personality."

The best cook in the house, hands down, was Jack, who was amazing and cooked every night. We were all annoyed when Jack got kicked off because none of the rest of us could cook. Bob's effort resulted in a 10-foot-tall grease fire in the kitchen. We went from eating lobster and steak to eating cereal.

The guys played a ton of hoops. Bob couldn't run because of a ruptured Achilles tendon, so he was always on my team. We played two-on-two with Charlie, Greg, Russ, or Rob, and had lots of tournaments. Bob's not the best hoops player, but he's disruptive to play against because he is always trash-talking. It worked out well that we played together . . . he annoyed the other team and I got to shoot. One day, Trista came over to say "Hi" before a date she was going on, and we just kept playing. In retrospect, we probably should have put the game on hold and said "Hello."

Then there was the attempted beach kiss. What a disaster! I call it the "diss kiss," a great TV moment. I had walked down the beach by myself, awaiting my turn to talk to Trista. I was worn down from the lack of sleep and the excess of partying, both of which are bad for anxiety, but I didn't want that to be an excuse. Today, I just wanted to be like everyone else. Beforehand, the producers had asked if any of us planned to kiss Trista. I said I'd try, but I was pretty sure she wouldn't kiss me back. We hadn't made much of a romantic connection. Still, I didn't mind the thought.

So when I finished talking to Trista at the beach, I asked if I could kiss her. It was just a little good night kiss, but it appeared extremely awkward, like the shower scene. She said I could kiss her on the cheek, and I did . . . fully realizing that America was going to watch me get shot down.

Then I went to my room and beat myself up for the stupid things I said and did, and . . . No! That's not what happened at all! Sure, it was embarrassing, but I was neither going to dwell on it nor play it over in my mind again and again so I could castigate myself for my ineptitude. I was human, not all of life is perfect, and I took a risk. So there.

These guys all had their own foibles and problems. Everyone in the world did, I realized. There's not a single person who gets to cruise through life like Joe Cool every day, with no little embarrassments, no skeletons in the closet. And if anxiety was my skeleton, well, I was taking it out of the closet. It could hold no more shame for me.

Panic was one part of who I was, and it turned out to be the thing I was most proud of. Until the show, I had still told only a handful of people about my struggles, but that was about to end. I confided in some of the guys in the house, and even the producers, as I worked my way up to admitting in front of the camera that I had this disorder.

■ ■ ■

Unless your family and friends have experienced social anxiety in some fashion, they are unlikely to understand the depths of your distress or know how to help you. Many people tend to associate social anxiety with shyness, which they tend to dismiss as a very common, minor, and temporary problem. Also, in our Western culture, we tend to expect and reward cheerfulness in the face of adversity, so people may tell you just to "cheer up" and get over it. This dismisses your apprehension, fear, dread, insecurity, uncertainty, embarrassment, and loss of dignity as a result. Moreover, this attitude makes it doubly difficult for you. You are saddled not only with the disorder but also with other people's judgments about whether you are handling your condition "appropriately." This is the last thing you need!

Understand that they are not being purposely unkind or callous, but it is imperative that you not allow yourself to feel bad about the situation if you get a reaction that's lacking in empathy. You did not create your problem and have little control over how others respond to it. Furthermore, how they feel is not a reflection of you or your condition.

You can choose to help them better understand your situation by explaining how your anxiety is a very real problem for you. Introducing the topic a little at a time can be useful. Letting it all hang out at once can be overwhelming. You need to focus the discussion on what your anxious thoughts and behaviors are and how they generally affect different aspects of your life. Leave the psychiatric labels at home.

—Signe Dayhoff, Ph.D.

■ ■ ■

I became desensitized to the cameras as time went on. The producers held daily interviews called ITMs ("in the moment"), and we each did two or three hourlong interviews a day. They base the shows around those interviews. My first few were difficult, and I stuck to short sentences. But soon, I wasn't fazed anymore. I learned to really enjoy the camera and let it spur me on—to come alive in its presence.

The TV show *EXTRA* came to interview us while we were filming, and they told me that I did a great job and came off as very poised and relaxed. They even had me do some reporting later. They told me I could make a good reporter, but ultimately ended up hiring Charlie full-time. (That guy is always beating me out!)

It felt great to hear those compliments because I wasn't sure how I did. We often see ourselves differently from the way that others see us. Those with social anxiety are prone to perceive themselves negatively, and those perceptions are usually not true.

It was really the host, Chris Harrison, who encouraged me to come forward about my panic attacks. On the reunion show, in front of a live audience and millions of at-home viewers, I sat in the hot seat and told the world that I had panic disorder and that I viewed it as a strength. A huge weight lifted from my shoulders as the words came out.

When I got dumped after the third round, I did feel a slight bit rejected. It's only natural, even though I knew we weren't right for each other. I was able to use it to get sympathy, though, when I told people that I was weeks away from getting engaged when the girl I had been dating dropped me for another guy.

Ryan and Trista proved to me that you can, in fact, find love anywhere. I was—and am—very happy for them, and so honored to be included at their wedding.

I think the television audience felt it was strange that so many of Trista's "exes" were there and that Charlie was hosting, but it wasn't strange for us. These weren't exactly long-term romances, and Ryan didn't feel threatened by any of the guys. He said afterward that we were all such good friends that it overshadowed the fact that we went on a couple of dates with Trista.

I sat at the wedding with Cowboy Brook, Angelique, and Shannon from *The Bachelor 1* and realized this thing was for real! Despite the helicopters and the $4 million budget, and the fact that I briefly honestly thought their wedding minister was Pierce Brosnan, this was a very real wedding that united two people who are deeply in love.

When country singer Brad Paisley sang Ryan's poem, I even got teary-eyed. Hey, don't give me that "sissy" look—everyone in the room got a little choked up. I went on to do some crazy dancing at the wedding, and thankfully, that didn't air. If there's anyone out there who can teach me to dance, call me! I need help!

After *The Bachelorette*, I got an e-mail from Quincy. We hadn't spoken in years, but a friend pointed her way to my Web site and she dropped me a sweet note to tell me it was fun to see me on TV. I went to visit her last March, and finally told her the truth about all I had been going through at college. We've been in touch ever since then.

■ ■ ■

I thought we'd meet for a quick drink, and five hours later, he had told me everything. He opened up about his anxiety disorder, and how he had really liked me and just couldn't bear to be with me because he would get so uncontrollably nervous. He said that when I would call and leave messages, he would have panic attacks just thinking about calling me back. I was shocked! In a way I was so happy and relieved that it wasn't me—it was what he was going through. But I wish I had known. Maybe I could've done something to help, maybe things would've gone differently. It's so great getting back in touch with him, though.

—Quincy Hentzel (high school girlfriend)

■ ■ ■

Being recognized was another experience that took some getting used to. Right after the first show aired, I went out to dinner with friends. When I looked up, people were staring at me and taking pictures. My motor skills vanished and the fork kept missing my mouth. But I soon got used to people recognizing me and knowing things about me. It was a massive dose of exposure therapy, and it wound up being so rewarding that it inspired this book.

The vast majority of feedback I've gotten from *The Bachelorette* has been tremendously positive, but sometimes it's been a bigger kick to eavesdrop on the more heated discussions about the show. While the show was airing, I was out to lunch and overheard four ladies chatting animatedly about it. When the talk turned to me, my ears perked up. They went around the table expressing their opinions about me, as if they'd known me for years. Two of them liked me, one thought I was okay, and the last one despised me.

The latter woman made fun of my blindingly, frighteningly white teeth and said I was a wimp for not making out with Trista in the shower and for asking for that good night kiss. Then another lady chimed in to agree.

"Yeah, now that I think about it, his face is a bit too long and his teeth are too big and white, and he looks like a Ken doll or an android or something," she said.

I was incognito in my sunglasses and hat and laughing out loud with one of my buddies. I turned around to join in their conversation and proceeded to rip on myself ruthlessly: "I met that guy, and he's as big a dork in person as he looks on TV. He has the personality of a pile of logs."

They were very interested in my opinion, so I continued to tell them, "Yes, he does look like an android, and he's fairly stupid. What kind of loser would go on a show like that anyway?"

They agreed, and said you'd have to be pretty desperate and pathetic. The kicker was when a fan recognized me despite the shades and hat and asked, "Are you Jamie from *The Bachelorette*? Can I take my picture with you?"

I said, "Sure," then walked away and smiled for the camera. I glanced back at the table, and all four ladies sat with their mouths wide open. The one who ripped on me ran over to apologize, and I told her not to worry about it. I told her I would think the same things she did. I was just saying that to put her at ease, but it occurred to me that at one time I really did think all those negative things about myself.

People come up to me all the time now, usually to share their stories about anxiety or ask for help. I was shooting baskets at a local gym when a father walked up to me with his boy and whispered, "I've got what you've got." I immediately knew what he meant. I asked if he wanted to talk in private, and he said yes. He looked so ashamed as he told me about his first panic attack. Here he was, a wealthy attorney with a great family and a nice house in the suburbs, and he was no more immune to panic attacks than I had been at 19. I could tell that the man had never really talked about his condition, and he was desperately afraid of the next time an attack would strike. I gave him some advice and told him which books to read. And I told him to call me anytime.

But one girl, in particular, made me realize that I had done the right thing by coming forward about my disorder. I was speaking and signing autographs in Orlando when a 14-year-old girl came up to me, shaking. She had been waiting in line to talk to me, and I thought she just really liked the show. But then she told me that she had been dealing with panic attacks at school and the kids had made fun of her ruthlessly. Her class was on a field trip to the function where I was speaking.

"When you told your story, it was the first time people understood what I've been going through," she said, and started to sob. For the first time, she wasn't alone in this.

Prior to that talk, I had doubts in my mind about whether or not I should have come out and told the world about my struggles with anxiety. Would it affect my future and what others thought about me? That girl erased all those doubts from my mind, and people like her the world over have made every day of struggle worthwhile.

I'm thankful to share my story and feel blessed that *The Bachelorette* gave me a chance to show the world that anxiety doesn't have to get the last laugh.

⋅⋅ 14 ⋅⋅

Ever After

Everything is possible for him who believes.
—MARK 9:23

I really didn't know which guy ended up with Trista until the rest of the world found out. Well, the truth is that I had a pretty good hunch, but I was in suspense for those last few shows too. We finished taping in mid-November, but the show's first episode wasn't televised until January 8.

In February, after the airing of the show where Trista and I said our goodbyes, I wrote this in my journal:

I am in NYC for the first time and staying in the luxurious Millennium Hotel, 40 stories up, overlooking the lights and action and vibrant energy of Times Square. In just six hours, I will be doing my first TV interview and it is with Diane Sawyer of Good Morning America . . . *live, I might add! I can't believe this is actually happening.*

If only Diane knew that the last time I saw her, she was giving a rousing speech at my graduation, where I was so downtrodden that in my wildest fantasies I couldn't imagine a day like this. It meant so much to me to be speaking with her.

I would do seven interviews that day, but *Good Morning America* was the first. And it seemed appropriate that I chose to talk publicly about my struggles with anxiety for the first time on Diane's show, because even though she had no idea at the time, she had a starring role on one of my hardest days. Although we had taped *The Bachelorette*'s reunion show, it hadn't yet aired, so I didn't have to mention anxiety on *Good Morning America*. No one would have asked me about it because no one knew about it. I could have just let the issue drop, but it felt too important now.

I knew I was going to bring it up, if given the chance, and that all of my friends and past coworkers—anyone who ever knew me— might be watching and judging me for it. But I had spent nine years hiding it. It was time to tell the truth and possibly help someone who was watching and feeling as low as I had.

Diane made it easy. She has a talent for making people feel important and comfortable, and I felt like we were just having a conversation with no one else around. The mask had been lifted and I liked the outlook. I walked off that stage with Bob Guiney, feeling confident and thankful.

Bob and I were a package deal that day, partially because we got booted off on the same episode, and partially because we hung out together so much on the show. Even though I had told Bob about my struggles, he still had trouble believing that things were as bad as I said they were. I took that as a great compliment: it meant that my anxiety didn't show.

Exiting our limo and en route to CNN for an interview with Connie Chung, I asked Bob, "What was she on before CNN?"

He replied, "You should tell her she was great in *Charlie's Angels*."

"Yeah, yeah, thanks Bob . . . wait, she wasn't on that . . . was she?"

"No, you goofball, she was on *The View* . . . you know, that morning talk show on ABC."

Tending to be somewhat gullible, I greeted Connie with, "You were great on *The View*!" She looked at me for a few seconds as if I were completely bananas and then she broke down in a fit of laughter, thinking that I intended this buffoon-like remark as a joke. Thanks, Bob.

Connie was very funny and laid-back and started the segment by interviewing Bob. He tends to ramble, so I wandered off in my head, kicking myself for telling her she was great on *The View*. She suddenly cut to me and said, "What do you think of that, Jamie?"

Lost in a daydream and having no idea what Bob had just said, I stammered, "Uh . . . um . . . um . . . is this thing live?"

Connie and Bob laughed like crazy, but I was just beginning my train-wreck-like behavior.

We met Vince Neil of Motley Crue in the green room of *The Caroline Rhea Show*, and I said, "I love your song 'Every Rose Has Its Thorn.'" Vince told me that was Poison.

Yeah, it was an entertaining day, and I was still on a high from the big truth-telling I'd done earlier. As I went to bed that night, I realized what a monumental thing I'd just done. No more secrets. No more shame. I had just gone from one extreme to another. I hadn't even told my old coworkers or most of my friends about my anxiety disorder before this, but now I had told the world and there was no turning back.

Reactions were astounding. Newspapers and magazines sent reporters to talk with me, radio shows called, and I felt like a poster boy for panic disorder. Most of the headlines were a variation of "He didn't get the girl, but he got his confidence back." I felt sheepish whenever approaching a newsstand . . . my picture was everywhere!

It seemed half the world came out of the woodwork to tell me about their anxiety disorders. People who worked with me in sales cried on my parents' answering machine, saying they had panic attacks too and wished I had told them what I was going through. Right after *The Bachelorette* ended, Charlie dated a woman who had panic disorder, and he told me that after seeing firsthand what a panic attack was like and how uncontrollable it can be, he was amazed by how far I'd come.

The talk shows and I got flooded with mail from people who were so happy to see a "success case." I prayed that I wouldn't let them down. It gave me an extra sense of responsibility to know that people were looking at me with hope in their eyes, expecting me to be bulletproof against anxiety now.

Sometimes it's harder for men to admit their fears; so many of the men who wrote were particularly glad that I spoke publicly about my problem. Often, men feel extra pressure to be "strong," and we believe that having a psychological problem somehow makes us less macho. We're allowed to break an arm or tear a ligament, but we're never supposed to feel scared or depressed or out of control.

Of course that's ridiculous, and as the letters poured in, I felt proud that I was standing up to the stigma. I hoped that if I had seen a guy like me on television when I was still suffering badly, I would have felt less ashamed and less alone.

Then Oprah Winfrey called to ask me to talk about my struggles with anxiety on her show. My brothers used to make fun of me because when I was going through panic and they wanted to watch *SportsCenter*, I was watching *Oprah*. She always had people on her show who had overcome obstacles, and the show gave me hope. So sure, the anxiety popped up before the limo came to get me.

When the negative thoughts crept in, I told myself, "All right, I'm nervous. I should be. Anybody would be—it's Oprah! But she is a human being like everyone else, and I've been on a dozen TV shows already and have done well. I'm going to expect panic to come and I know how to deal with it. I am more prepared than I have ever been. I deserve to do well and I will."

So, no, I'm not bulletproof. I don't suppose anyone is. But that isn't the important part. The important part is to keep setting your sights higher in defiance of that anxiety. If it visits again, keep slamming the door in its face until it takes a hint: you're not going to bow down to its bullying techniques. You're going to live your life anyway.

And that's what I did. I sat there with Oprah—and other people who went through anxiety disorders, including NFL star Ricky Williams—and I talked about my terror, my suicidal thoughts, my breakdown. Just by talking about it, by throwing it out there in the open and refusing to be ashamed anymore, I had taken away another piece of the panic's power over me.

Oprah's staff told me the response to the show was outstanding, and they sent me some of the mail viewers wrote to me. I couldn't stop smiling when I saw how many people were inspired by our stories and asked for a follow-up show.

■ ■ ■

It has helped immensely to know that there are men who suffer from this. It also helps to know that it can be overcome. The show gave me so much courage and drive to try to do something about this. This may sound corny, but the next time I feel the anxiety (which will likely be today) I will think about the show and the words you spoke about confronting it and knowing that I can get through it.

Thanks, Jamie. You have become a bit of a role model, and I appreciate your honesty and strength.

—From an e-mail Jamie received after
The Oprah Winfrey Show

■ ■ ■

Over the months to come, I did countless interviews on television, radio, and in print, and I got to meet people from other seasons of *The Bachelor* and *The Bachelorette* when we got together in places like Las Vegas for reunions. I also got to meet the women from *The Bachelor 4* when I made a guest appearance to help Bob narrow down the field. Boy, was I envious! These women had it all. It was a blast meeting them. And with all the pressure off me, I was able to relax and have a great time on the show.

I'm still friends with many people from the series—Charlie, Bob, Greg, Jack, Rob, Brook, Russ, Ryan, Trista, Shannon, Tina Fabulous, Estella, Kelly Jo, Angelique, Gwen, Helene, and the host, Chris Harrison, who was one of the funniest guys in the bunch (which you'd never know based on his hosting persona). He used to hang out with us at the bachelor pad and play pool with us. I later went to visit Chris and his cool wife Gwen, and Chris woke me up by saying, "Jamie, you can say your goodbyes!" just like he says on the show. As I'm writing this, I just came back from a trip where a bunch of us from the show visited Ryan and Trista and went snowboarding. I'm doubly thankful to ABC for giving me a chance to become friends with all these people whom I never would have otherwise met.

One of the great things about being recognizable is that you get to meet so many interesting and nice people who will open up to you because they feel they've gotten to know you—after all, you've been making weekly appearances in their living rooms. And for a brief time, I got a cool glimpse into the life of a star—riding in limos everywhere I went, room service, five-star hotels in the Caribbean, Vegas, Miami, Palm Springs, New York City . . . all places I had never been to before.

The dichotomy of that glamorous life and the lives of my Little League team, which I still coach by the way, is sometimes hard to reconcile. The kids live about a 10-minute drive to Lake Michigan and yet only one or two of them has seen it. None of them have traveled outside of Chicago. They have never seen a mountain or an ocean or anything outside of their current reality. I saw success happen in these kids because Brian Musso and I took an interest in them.

Have you ever seen a flea circus? Okay, probably not, but if you wonder how people "train" fleas, it's pretty simple. You put them in a jar with a lid on. For a while, they'll jump like crazy and hit their heads on the lid, but then they'll adjust their jumps and stay within the limits of the jar. When you take the lid off, they will stay put and not jump out. In fact, you can take them out of the jar entirely and they'll just jump in place as if they were still imprisoned. They have been conditioned to their surroundings. Sometimes we just set our sights too low and forget about our potential.

We need to stretch ourselves beyond our comfort zone and beyond our current realities to discover our full potential. It was true for these kids, and it's true for everyone out there who has an anxiety disorder. The goal was to get them to realize that, as hard as their lives were, they could not make themselves victims. If they had the right attitude and work ethic, they could be successes despite their challenging environment.

They needed to know the things that determine success or failure. Then they needed to learn that they could be in control of them. They could control their attitudes, beliefs, and effort. The goal was to instill the habits that would lead to an overall increase in their self-esteem. First, we had to inspire them to look beyond their current reality. Then we had to instill the attitudes, knowledge, and skills that are necessary both in playing baseball and in life. It's done with hard work and focus and repetition.

The first day, we met a dozen 9- to 12-year-olds on a lousy little field. At least, they were supposed to be 9 to 12, but about half of them were younger and had just lied on their application forms. I asked, "How many of you have played baseball?" No hands went up. They didn't know how to hold a ball or a bat. I asked who wanted to play catcher, and they didn't know what the positions were. It was like they had grown up on Mars. And they were looking at me like I was an alien.

They were slouched over and talking together, some making fun of me. But at the same time, they were curious. They were used to people, especially authority figures, making promises to them and not following through. I now understood that the most important thing was just to show up, as Bob Muzikowski had taught me when I first started coaching Little League.

We worked on the basics of fielding a groundball . . . over and over and over. We had a kid named Terrence, whose attitude was less than spectacular the first year. But because of all the practice we did, going over and over the fundamentals of fielding a groundball, this kid came back the next year as the best fielder on the team, with an improved attitude. He used to strike out or commit an error and then erupt in rage and get thrown out of the game. He didn't get thrown out of one game the second year and was by far the most improved player on the team. As I had learned in conquering my panic, we needed to bring out these kids' hidden potential and cultivate positive attitudes.

∎ ∎ ∎

Jamie's great with these kids because he can go back now to that funny guy he was in high school, and it makes the kids laugh. He has a gift to be able to do that. They really connect with him because he can get right on their level.

—Brian Musso

∎ ∎ ∎

We had 15 games the first year. We lost our first 7 by the "slaughter rule"—the games were stopped early because we were being trounced so badly. When a couple of runs were scored against them, they'd want to give up; they'd get down on each other. I worked hard to catch them doing something right. I rewarded positive effort, attitude, and teamwork, regardless of wins or losses.

Now it was our eighth game, against the best team in the league, last inning. Our pitcher was facing their best batter, with two outs. He struck him out—and he ran into my arms, crying with jubilation. The team went nuts. We won our last eight games, to finish 8 and 7.

It was a good example in a microcosm of what is possible. The result was that the kids started to believe in themselves. The by-product was that they won baseball games, but the larger effect was that they began thinking about what could be possible outside of the projects. The same can be true of anxiety—maybe beating your anxiety will just be a by-product, and the real effect will be that your life becomes more joyful and filled with possibility and reignited dreams once the limits are lifted.

■ ■ ■

Adversity and difficult situations are lessons designed for personal growth, not random and capricious acts of fate. If you accept the idea that life is a classroom, then having to contend with an anxiety disorder (or any other difficult malady) is part of the curriculum. You can gain considerable strength, character, and compassion from working with and striving to overcome your difficulties.

—Edmund J. Bourne, Ph.D.

■ ■ ■

One of my own dreams is yet to be realized. I'm still single and searching for my match. My dating life has been more active these days, but love hasn't hit me over the head yet. I'm hoping to find someone who is outgoing and sociable, enthusiastic about life, kind of quirky—motivated to achieve her goals, but funny and maybe a little goofy.

Even though I haven't found romantic love yet, the love of my family and friends always sustains me. I wish everyone who has an anxiety disorder has the kind of supportive people around him or her that I have. I honestly don't know what I would have done if not for their care and dedication.

Once the show mania died down, I again wondered what I'd do with my life next. But it wasn't a desperate, worried feeling anymore—now the world was alive with possibility, and I could pick and choose my next path. I took on some guest reporting jobs for ABC in Chicago and Portland, spoke at the Anxiety Disorders

Association of America's annual conference, played basketball again, and honed my public speaking skills all across North America by giving speeches about anxiety disorders. I really enjoyed reporting and hope to do more of it in the future. In the meantime, I had one major goal still to be fulfilled: I wanted to write a book.

Although it had been a vague notion before—I knew I wanted to write a book, but I didn't know what I would write about—now I had a real reason to write one. I remembered how hopeless and alone and crazy I felt when I was locked into my dorm room and wishing the world would disappear. I read the thousands of e-mails from people who wrote to tell me about their own difficulties with anxiety. Strangers cried in my arms, so relieved to find that someone in the world understood what they were going through.

I'm a regular guy who got a taste of fame for no real reason. When Tina Fabulous and I did an appearance in Miami, people crowded us as we got out of the limo and asked what we were doing in town. "We're here to film *Barbie and Ken, the Movie*," I joked—and people believed it. Before the show, nobody cared who I was, and I didn't earn fame through special talents like acting or singing. I just went on camera and acted kind of like myself. I still couldn't believe people wanted my autograph. But this measure of fame gave me a megaphone to shout to the world that there is always hope. If I was going to get only 15 minutes of fame, I was going to use that time to help people.

■ ■ ■

I am a 50-something schoolteacher who has suffered from constant panic disorder and occasional social phobia for many, many years. When I saw you on *The Oprah Show*, it was like God sent you to speak directly to me. I thought to myself, if this handsome young man can struggle for years with panic and social anxiety disorder and overcome it, then

I also can overcome my problems. Many times I did not attend weddings, birthday parties, or family outings because I was afraid. I now have HOPE, and I never had that before seeing you on TV.

—From an e-mail Jamie received

■ ■ ■

Beating anxiety and depression takes a battle; that's for sure. But it's a battle that's worth it, because in the end you get your life back. I'm not superhuman—if I can do it, you can.

Recently, I talked to Grant, my friend from sales, and he asked me, "Do you remember when I asked you what you were going to do now that you had quit and were out of a job? You told me that you were going to play pro hoops, get on a TV show, and then write a book. I'm proud of you, buddy, and I didn't believe you. I thought you were crazy. You still are crazy, though."

Maybe so. A little bit crazy, a little eccentric. I hear that Pearl Jam song "Alive" these days and I remember that, just a few years ago, I didn't know how I was going to survive. Today, I've done far better than survive. I'm living a life worth living.

■ ■ ■

What Jamie has done is extraordinary. He was obviously very motivated to do these things and has, as a consequence, proved something to himself and others. While everyone needs to have goals she or he wants to fulfill, those goals do not have to be audacious like Jamie's. They can be big or small or somewhere in between. What these goals should reflect is what each individual personally wants to make his or her life truly satisfying.

—Signe Dayhoff, Ph.D.

■ ■ ■

My life—my real life—started with my first panic attack. Now, when I look back on my days mired in suffering, I feel a surge of relief wash over me. I nearly didn't make it . . . but would I rewrite my life's script? If I could go back and change history so I never went through social anxiety and panic disorder, would I?

Not a chance.

Friedrich Nietzsche wrote something that has become a cliché: "What does not destroy me, makes me stronger." It's a cliché because it's true: my anxiety disorder was the toughest thing I've ever had to overcome, but in the process, I had to face all of the things that had ever scared me and held me back. I had to challenge myself to become tougher and more self-confident, and I had to put a tremendous amount of faith in myself for the first time.

I will never forget my fear. Thank God for that, because I don't ever want to. It's not something I now see as shameful. Quite the opposite: I am so proud that I stood tall against this adversary and chose to go through all the trials to get to where I am now. Pain is temporary, but quitting and avoidance last forever. In my battle, I found strengths and abilities I never knew I had. It shaped me into a better man, and for that, I am grateful.

I can't tell you how strange it feels for me to write an ending to a book on overcoming anxiety. I wish I could go back into that bare dorm room and tap that shaking kid on the shoulder and reassure him that there was joy to be found on the other side of all that fear. That life could still be a beautiful and exciting adventure, and that his dreams didn't have to shrivel up and die. I can't, but I can tell you. Maybe you're that same kid, or maybe you know someone just like him. If you do, I hope you'll share this message.

If you are feeling hopeless, trapped in a mind swirling with doubts and insecurities, I want to tell you without hesitation that you can rise above it and live a happy and fulfilled life. Panic seemed to me like a wall that was insurmountable—I couldn't see past it, and I certainly didn't think I had the endurance to climb over it. No matter what your obstacle is—whether it's anxiety or anything else—I want to implore you to fight to excavate the courage that you have stored deep inside.

Ignite that spark and act on it today. Unwrap the present of your life each day. This moment is a moment to change your life for the better. Never settle for your life because you're used to it or because the fight seems too hard. Your expectations don't need to be lowered by anxiety. History gives us example after example of people who have succeeded despite all odds.

After he beat brain cancer, Lance Armstrong won six straight Tours de France—something he was never able to do before the cancer.

Jackie Robinson carried the weight of the world on his shoulders when he broke the color barrier in major league baseball. He received death threats and racist slurs and got knocked down time and again by pitchers who threw the ball at his head, but he kept dusting himself off and following his heart. If he failed, he felt he was failing African Americans everywhere. Now that's pressure!

He became a six-time All Star and was inducted into the Baseball Hall of Fame, even though his wife worried that he was having a nervous breakdown in the process. He once said, "Life is not a spectator sport. If you're going to spend your whole life in the grandstands just watching what goes on, in my opinion you're wasting your life."

■ ■ ■

This is not an accident. People who suffer from chronic anxiety in any of its terrible forms learn to be heroes. If you want a hero, look for someone who is terrified.

—Bob Rich, Ph.D.

■ ■ ■

And what about you? What will you choose to do with your life? Whatever obstacles stand in your way, you have the power to move them out of the way. I can't tell you that it'll be easy, but I can tell you that you are worth the fight, no matter how long it takes or how hard it gets.

There is no shame in seeking help. To find a therapist, a good place to start is the Anxiety Disorders Association of America (they maintain a directory of anxiety specialists at www.adaa.org, searchable by city or zip code), or equivalent associations in other countries (like the Anxiety Disorders Association of Canada). You can also check at local teaching hospitals to see whether they have anxiety specialty clinics and ask your family doctor for recommendations.

■ ■ ■

The main thing is to find a therapist who is familiar with evidence-based treatments for anxiety disorders such as cognitive behavioral treatments or medications. Look for people who have experience with your specific type of anxiety disorder. And if you don't feel improvement within a few months, find a new therapist.

Most people start to make gains within six weeks or so of treatment. The typical treatment using cognitive behavioral therapy lasts about 12 sessions in the course of 14 to 16 weeks. Some people get to the point at the end of the three or four months where anxiety is not an issue at all anymore, and some people still struggle with it and, ideally, continue to work on it and continue to improve after the end of treatment. I would say 75 to 80 percent of people make some improvement in therapy. A lot of people reach a point where it's no longer interfering with their life and it's not an issue anymore. Their anxiety is in the normal range.

—Martin Antony, Ph.D.

■ ■ ■

If you're going to stand up to anxiety, the first thing you need is faith, because it may take some time for you to see evidence that you're recovering. Sometimes other people can see we're getting better before we realize it ourselves. When doubts creep in, stick to your plan and envision the positive future that awaits you if you just hang in there five minutes longer.

Do something small today that's a challenge for you, whether that's going out to the mall, driving one block, starting a thought journal, making an appointment to see a therapist, or calling a friend and telling the truth about why you haven't been "yourself" lately. Take on another challenge tomorrow, and the next day. Repeat challenges until you feel you've mastered them, and don't feel bad if it takes more time than you think it "should." Every time you try is an achievement in itself. Every time you try to do something that anxiety wants to stop you from doing, you've struck a blow that will make the anxiety weaker. It may hit you back, but you're the one with the stamina. Hang in there and watch as that boxer loses steam. You won't know which blow has delivered the knockout punch until you get there.

The shadows will pass if you choose to fight. Choose to speak up for yourself when fear tells you that you can't do it. Get up every day with hope in your heart no matter how grim it seems and let the pain lead you to carve out a worthy life that's bigger and grander than you ever imagined before. In doing so, you win.

We all have a time when our backs are against the wall, when we are staring into the abyss, when there is no one to lean on but our own wounded spirits. I had my time, and someday my strength will be tested again. Thunderbolts crash down, and with them come doubt, fear, and hopelessness.

That is when you need to believe, to have faith when all of the signs say it's impossible. Even a wounded spirit can crush its captor. You'll find your way out, and it probably won't look exactly like my way or anyone else's way. Listen to the people who've shared your struggle, take from us whatever you can, and don't be afraid to make up your own rules to fill in the rest.

It's time for you to believe in your own inherent power. Victory is more than just a TV show or a sales call or a date or a public talk. It's about being the underdog, about giving it your best shot despite the seemingly overwhelming obstacles, despite the pain. Know that you are an important person and your life matters.

Let's fight together and for each other. Let's throw away the shame and talk to one another without the facades so we can all know that none of us is ever alone. Pain may unite us today, but triumph can be our everlasting prize if we help one another find our way out of the darkness.

Resources

Below are organizations, Web sites, and books I hope you will find useful in your journey.

ORGANIZATIONS

ANXIETY DISORDERS ASSOCIATION OF AMERICA (ADAA)

8730 Georgia Avenue, Suite 600
Silver Spring, MD 20910
(240) 485-1001
www.adaa.org
(Includes a list of support groups organized by state, as well as anxiety treatment providers searchable by zip code.)

CENTER FOR HELP FOR ANXIETY/AGORAPHOBIA THROUGH NEW GROWTH EXPERIENCES (CHAANGE)

1360 Rosecrans Street, Suite I
San Diego, CA 92106
(619) 224-2216
www.chaange.com

CLINICAL RESEARCH UNIT FOR ANXIETY AND DEPRESSION (CRUFAD)
CRUFAD at St Vincent's Hospital
299 Forbes Street
Darlinghurst, Sydney
NSW, 2010
Australia
www.crufad.com/cru_index.htm

NATIONAL ALLIANCE FOR THE MENTALLY ILL (NAMI)
Colonial Place Three
2107 Wilson Boulevard, Suite 300
Arlington, VA 22201-3042
(800) 950-6264
www.nami.org

NATIONAL INSTITUTE OF MENTAL HEALTH (NIMH)
6001 Executive Boulevard, Rm. 8184 MSC 9663
Bethesda, MD 20892-9663
(888) 8-ANXIETY
www.nimh.nih.gov/anxiety/anxiety/index.htm

TOASTMASTERS INTERNATIONAL
P.O. Box 9052
Mission Viejo, CA 92690
(949) 858-8255
www.toastmasters.org

WEB SITES

ANXIETY DISORDERS INFORMATION AND RESOURCES
www.mental-health-matters.com/disorders/dis_category.php?
catID=10

THE ANXIETY PANIC INTERNET RESOURCE
www.algy.com/anxiety/

ENCOURAGE CONNECTION
www.encourageconnection.com

PANIC/ANXIETY DISORDERS
www.panicdisorder.about.com

SUGGESTED READING

Anger and Anxiety by Bob Rich, Ph.D. (North Charleston, SC:
Booksurge, 2002)

The Anxiety and Phobia Workbook by Edmund Bourne (Oakland,
CA: New Harbinger, revised in 2001)

Beyond Shyness: How to Conquer Social Anxieties by Jonathan Berent
with Amy Lemley (New York: Simon & Schuster, 1993)

Conquering Panic and Anxiety Disorders, edited by Jenna Glatzer
with Paul Foxman, Ph.D. (Alameda, CA: Hunter House, 2002)

*Dancing with Fear: Overcoming Anxiety in a World of Stress and
Uncertainty* by Paul Foxman, Ph.D. (Lanham, MD: Rowman &
Littlefield Publishers, Inc., 2002)

Diagonally-Parked in a Parallel Universe: Working Through Social Anxiety by Signe A. Dayhoff (Placitas, NM: Effectiveness-Plus Publications, 2000)

Dying of Embarrassment: Help for Social Anxiety and Phobia by C. Alec Pollard, Ph.D., Barbara G. Markway, Ph.D., Cheryl N. Carmin, and Teresa Flynn (Oakland, CA: New Harbinger, 1992)

Painfully Shy: How to Master Social Anxiety and Reclaim Your Life by Barbara G. Markway, Ph.D., and Gregory P. Markway, Ph.D. (New York: St. Martin's Press, 2003)

The Shyness and Social Anxiety Workbook by Martin Antony, Ph.D. (Oakland, CA: New Harbinger, 2000)

Triumph Over Fear: A Book of Help and Hope for People with Anxiety, Panic Attacks, and Phobias by Jerilyn Ross (New York: Bantam Doubleday Dell Publishing Group, 1995)

About the Contributors

MARTIN M. ANTONY, PH.D., is professor in the Department of Psychiatry and Behavioural Neurosciences at McMaster University. He is also chief psychologist and director of the Anxiety Treatment and Research Centre at St. Joseph's Healthcare in Hamilton, Ontario. Dr. Antony has published 11 books and more than 80 scientific articles and book chapters in the areas of anxiety disorders and cognitive behavior therapy. His work has been recognized by awards from the Society of Clinical Psychology (American Psychological Association), the Canadian Psychological Association, and the Anxiety Disorders Association of America. Dr. Antony's Web site can be found at www.martinantony.com.

JONATHAN BERENT, A.C.S.W., is the author of *Beyond Shyness: How to Conquer Social Anxieties* (Simon & Schuster, 1993). In private psychotherapy practice since 1978 in Great Neck, New York, he and his staff have treated thousands of individuals with social anxiety. Media experience includes interviews with Oprah Winfrey, Sally Jessy Raphael, Joan Rivers, CNN Medical News, CNBC, many network news programs, the *New York Times, Newsday, Readers Digest,* the *Boston Globe,* and many, many radio shows. Visit www.socialanxiety.com.

EUGENE BERESIN, M.D., is associate professor of psychiatry at Harvard Medical School in Boston, where he has served for more than 25 years. He's also the director of child and adolescent psychiatry training at Massachusetts General Hospital and McLean Hospital, a psychiatric facility that's a longstanding leader in the research and treatment of mental illness and chemical dependency.

EDMUND J. BOURNE, PH.D., has specialized in the treatment of anxiety disorders and related problems for two decades. For many years, he was director of The Anxiety Treatment Center in San Jose and Santa Rosa, California. His bestselling anxiety workbooks (all published by New Harbinger Publications), which have helped hundreds of thousands of people throughout the world, include *The Anxiety and Phobia Workbook* (revised 2001), *Beyond Anxiety and Phobia* (2001), and *Coping with Anxiety* (2003). His latest book is *Natural Relief for Anxiety* (2004). Dr. Bourne lives and practices in Hawaii and California.

SIGNE A. DAYHOFF, PH.D., M.A., M.ED., is a social psychologist with counseling training. Through her company, Effectiveness-Plus LLC, she provides social effectiveness coaching, training, and resources to alleviate social and performance anxiety and shyness, create high-octane self-confidence, and develop effective interpersonal and conversational skills. Her latest book is *Diagonally-Parked in a Parallel Universe: Working Through Social Anxiety* (Effectiveness-

Plus Publications, 2000), the social phobic's bible and positive life strategy approach. Her Web site is www.effectiveness-plus.com.

PAUL FOXMAN, PH.D., is in private practice specializing in the treatment of anxiety disorders, stress, and relationship problems. He has worked with adults, adolescents, and children for 25 years and is the director of the Center for Anxiety Disorders, a treatment program with office locations in Vermont, and regional coordinator and therapist trainer for Center for Help for Anxiety/Agoraphobia through New Growth Experiences (CHAANGE), a national anxiety treatment organization. He is the author of *Dancing with Fear* (Rowman & Littlefield, 1996), *The Worried Child* (Hunter House, 2004), *Conquering Panic and Anxiety Disorders* (Hunter House, 2003), and other publications, as well as a frequent presenter at professional conferences and expert on radio and television shows with a focus on stress and anxiety. Dr. Foxman received his B.A. in psychology from Yale University and his Ph.D. in clinical psychology from Vanderbilt University. He completed clinical training at the Department of Psychiatry, Mt. Zion Hospital, San Francisco, California, and the Kennedy Child Study Center, Nashville, Tennessee. He is a member of the American Psychological Association, Vermont Psychological Association, and National Register of Health Service Providers in Psychology. Visit www.drfoxman.com.

BARBARA G. MARKWAY, PH.D., is a psychologist, author, and founder of The Anxiety & Stress Management Center of Mid-Missouri in Jefferson City, Missouri. She is the coauthor of *Dying of Embarrassment: Help for Social Anxiety and Phobia* (New Harbinger, 1992) and *Painfully Shy: How to Master Social Anxiety and Reclaim Your Life* (St. Martin's Griffin, 2003). A sought-after expert, she has been a guest on *Good Morning America*, was featured in an award-winning documentary called *Afraid of People*, and has been

quoted in magazines such as *Prevention* and *Woman's World.* To
learn more about Dr. Markway or to contact her, visit her Web site
at www.painfullyshy.com.

GREGORY P. MARKWAY, PH.D., is a licensed clinical psychologist
practicing at St. Marys Health Center's Mental Health Services
in Jefferson City, Missouri. He has worked in the Behavioral
Medicine Department at the Washington University Medical
Center and was on the clinical faculty at the Washington University
School of Medicine.

CARRIE MASIA-WARNER, PH.D., is assistant professor of psychiatry
at the NYU School of Medicine and a member of the Institute of
Anxiety and Mood Disorders at the NYU Child Study Center. She
has authored and coauthored several articles on the assessment and
treatment of anxiety disorders in children and adolescents. Dr.
Masia-Warner received her B.A. degree in psychology from the
State University of New York at Binghamton. She received her
M.A. and Ph.D. in clinical psychology from West Virginia
University. Prior to joining the faculty at NYU, she completed a
two-year post-doctoral research fellowship in the Department of
Child Psychiatry at Columbia University, New York State
Psychiatric Institute.

HEIDI (REICHENBERGER) MCINDOO, M.S., R.D., L.D.N., is a nutrition
consultant specializing in nutrition education, communication,
and culinary topics. She received her B.S. in dietetics from the
University of Connecticut and her M.S. in nutrition communications from Tufts University. She spent four and a half years as a
clinical and outpatient dietitian at the Naval Submarine Base
Hospital in Connecticut. She also served as the head of the

Nutrition Department. While there, Ms. Reichenberger was awarded the Meritorious Civilian Service Medal by the Department of the Navy. She's a freelance writer whose work has been published in newspapers, magazines such as *Fitness*, cookbooks, and Web sites. She's also a national media spokesperson for the American Dietetic Association and has been quoted in several magazines and TV broadcasts.

C. ALEC POLLARD, PH.D., director of the Anxiety Disorders Center at the St. Louis Behavioral Medicine Institute and professor of community and family medicine at St. Louis University, is one of the nation's foremost authorities on social anxiety disorders. Between half and two-thirds of the patients treated in his intensive program come from outside St. Louis. His center treats patients with obsessive-compulsive disorder, panic, agoraphobia, post-traumatic stress disorders, and social anxiety disorders. Dr. Pollard is coauthor of *Dying of Embarrassment: Help for Social Anxiety and Phobia* (New Harbinger, 1992) and *The Agoraphobia Workbook: A Comprehensive Program to End Your Fear of Symptom Attacks* (New Harbinger, 2003).

BOB RICH, PH.D., is an Australian psychologist with more than 30 years of experience. People suffering from emotional or interpersonal problems can gain solace, advice, and help by visiting www.anxietyanddepression-help.com. Bob is also an author with 12 published books. Three of them have won international awards. Don't visit his writing showcase at www.bobswriting.com unless you have time to spend. People tend to get lost in his stories and book extracts.

About the Author

Jamie Blyth gained nationwide attention when he appeared as one of the final suitors on the ABC-TV reality series *The Bachelorette*. After going public with his nine-year-long battle with social anxiety disorder and panic attacks, he received tens of thousands of e-mails from fans who shared their own experiences of anxiety and fear. Blyth speaks for associations, including the Anxiety Disorders Association of America (ADAA), and universities around the country, and he has been a guest on *Oprah, Good Morning America,* and other national news programs and talk shows.